THE YELLOW EMPEROR'S
CLASSIC OF MEDICINE

THE
YELLOW
EMPEROR'S
CLASSIC
OF
MEDICINE

A New Translation of the NEIJING SUWEN

with Commentary

MAOSHING NI, PH.D.

SHAMBHALA
Boston and London
1995

Shambhala Publications, Inc.
Horticultural Hall
300 Massachusetts Avenue
Boston, Massachusetts 02115
http://www.shambhala.com

9   8   7   6   5   4   3   2

Printed in the United States of America
♾ This edition is printed on acid-free paper that meets the American National
Standards Institute Z39.48 Standard.
Distributed in the United States by Random House, Inc., and
in Canada by Random House of Canada Ltd

Library of Congress Cataloging-in-Publication Data
Su wen. English.
      The Yellow Emperor's Classic of medicine: a new translation
of the Neijing Suwen with commentary/Maoshing Ni.
—1st ed.
         p.   cm.
      Includes bibliographical references and index.
      ISBN 1-57062-080-6 (acid-free paper)
      1. Su wen.   2. Medicine, Chinese—Early works to 1800.
I. Ni, Maoshing.   II. Title.
R127.1.S93Y4513   1995   94-44058
610'.951—dc20   CIP

Dedicated to a world in need
of balance and harmony

CONTENTS

PREFACE

As the end of the twentieth century nears, humankind can celebrate the triumph of achievements in many fields, most notably science, technology, and medicine. The technological breakthroughs of the last two centuries that helped propel science to its zenith are responsible for raising standards of living, increasing productivity, and saving lives. Most significant is the increase in the communication of knowledge that made the vast application of science and technology possible. Paradoxically, the same accomplishments are also responsible for genocide on a massive scale, the destruction of our planet, and a gradual diminishing of quality in people's lives.

In recent years more and more disenchanted citizens of the West have looked to the East for an "organic" answer to the great imbalance in the technologically advanced "modern world." Strangely, few realize that the East, specifically China, contributed many discoveries and inventions to the modern world. According to Robert Temple in his book *The Genius of China,* some of the West's greatest achievements have turned out to be simple borrowing from the Chinese. These include decimal mathematics, paper and printing, the mechanical clock, guns, multistage rockets, the magnetic compass, a ship's rudder, manned flight, the steam engine, paper money, and even brandy and whiskey.

But the scientific and industrial revolutions did not occur in China, despite many advances prior to those of the West. One of the key reasons is that Chinese science and technology always functioned within a philosophy that recognized the importance of balance and harmony between human beings and the environment. In fact, there is more similarity between this philosophy-science paradigm of China and that of the ancient Greeks. As Joseph Needham, author of the great work *Science and Civilization in China,* wrote, "The sciences of China . . . never dreamed of divorcing science from ethics, but when at the Scientific Revolution the final cause of Aristotle was done away with, and ethics chased out of science, things became very different, and more menacing."

Without sensitive regard to the larger scheme of the universal law, modern science and technology will continue to produce disturbance and even destruction to all life on earth. In the modern age the East can indeed offer the West a philosophy of balance and harmony that is not only urgently needed but necessary for the survival of human civilization. No other Chinese source of this wisdom is as complete as the *Yellow Emperor's Classic of Medicine,* or the *Neijing.*

This monumental classic is undoubtedly the most important work representing the crowning achievement of the Chinese prior to the first unification of the country by Emperor Qin Shi in 221 BCE. Its authorship was attributed to the great Huang Di, the Yellow Emperor, who reigned during the middle of the third millennium BCE. The Chinese refer to themselves as the descendants of Huang Di, who is the symbol of the vital spirit of Chinese civilization. The *Neijing* is actually two works: the *Suwen* and the *Lingshu.* The *Suwen,* "Questions of Organic and Fundamental Nature," is the subject of this translation, while the *Lingshu,* once called *Zhen Jing,* or "Classic of Acupuncture," is a technical book on acupuncture and moxibustion.* Historically, *Neijing* refers to the *Suwen* alone.

I did not have full appreciation for the *Neijing* at an early age despite having been exposed to it through my father as well as through other Chinese classics. After an education and apprenticeship in Chinese medicine and philosophy I ventured on to study Western medicine, psychology, and physics. Through the Western sciences I gained an understanding for the pertinence of the wisdom outlined in this ancient classic. Furthermore, after I began my clinical practice of Chinese medicine, I became profoundly impressed by what the ancients had already understood thousands of years ago. The observations in the *Neijing* were stunningly scientific. Its contents are as relevant for life in the twentieth century as they were two millennia ago.

The *Neijing* of the Yellow Emperor is one of the most important classics of Taoism. First, it gives a holistic picture of human life. It does not separate external changes—geographic, climatic, and seasonal, for instance—from internal changes such as emotions and our responses to them. It tells how our way of life and our environment affect our health. Without going into fine detail, the *Neijing* articulates a treasure of ancient knowledge

---

*Moxibustion is a method of warming an acupuncture point by burning the herb mugwort over it.

concerning the natural way to health, implying that all phenomena of the
world stimulate, tonify, subdue, or depress one's natural life force. This
holistic life philosophy of the ancient developed ones represents the basic
tenets of the Integral Way—a life lived in harmony with the universal law.

The impact of the *Neijing* on subsequent Chinese discoveries and inventions is far-reaching. Its material is not confined merely to Chinese
medicine, though there is no higher authority than this; it also discusses all
the facets of human life that affect birth, growth, reproduction, and death.
In this significant work, one will find a wealth of knowledge—etiology,
physiology, diagnosis, therapy, and prevention of disease—as well as an in-
depth investigation of such diverse subjects as ethics, psychology, astronomy, meteorology, and chronobiology. All the subjects are discussed in a
holistic context that says life is not fragmented, as envisioned by modern
science, but rather that all the pieces make up an interconnected whole.
Humans are the offspring of the universe and therefore are subject to its
laws.

The *Neijing* offers much practical advice on how to maintain balance
by revealing the inner workings of the universal law. The environment,
the way of life, and the spirit all contribute to the quality of human existence. The essence of the *Neijing* can be summed up in the following passage: "Health and well-being can be achieved only by remaining centered
in spirit, guarding against the squandering of energy, promoting the constant flow of qi and blood, maintaining harmonious balance of yin and
yang, adapting to the changing seasonal and yearly macrocosmic influences,
and nourishing one's self preventively. This is the way to a long and happy
life."

The *Neijing* presents broad concepts and in many instances is brief
with details. When reading the *Neijing* there is much to be gained by understanding it from a perspective of openness as it generously shares the
wisdom imparted from an ancient tradition benefiting the health and lives
of humankind. The student and practitioner of Chinese medicine will be
amazed to find how little Chinese medicine has changed since the time the
Neijing was written. Its natural therapies and preventive approaches are
ever as effective and even more pertinent in today's drug-oriented medical
climate. It offers a heartfelt and viable approach in the perception and treatment of illness. Especially in the battle against chronic, degenerative, infectious, and deficient medical conditions, Chinese medicine is promising as

an effective alternative. The *Neijing*'s philosophy will help guide society in its pursuit of a higher quality of life.

Ironically, as China frantically races to industrialize, its citizens have lost sight of the Integral Way as expounded in the *Neijing*. Modernism at any cost to the internal as well as the external environment of humankind will no doubt create imbalances reflected in the health and the spirit of its people. With the ecological balance of our planet in peril, the message of the *Neijing* becomes even more significant. It speaks loud and clear: Degradation to our environment will have an irrevocable impact on all life on earth. On this point, Needham in *Science and Civilization in China* eloquently stated, "Science needs to be lived alongside religion, philosophy, history and aesthetic experience; alone it can lead to great harm." The *Neijing* offers a framework by which modern science, technology, and medicine can integrate with the natural principles of traditional Chinese medicine. This is the Integral Way. And this integration will, I hope, in the not-so-distant future, result in a more healthy, balanced, and harmonious existence for all people. This important book shows us that from the microcosm of human life we may learn the vast and profound realities of the macrocosm.

MAOSHING NI
Los Angeles
Spring 1994

A NOTE ON THE TRANSLATION

WHEN I first began my translation of the *Yellow Emperor's Classic of Medicine*, I was overwhelmed by its breadth of study and the complexity of the classical Chinese that was employed. As Ilze Veith pointed out in his own admirable translation of this text, the challenge lies in the fact that each classical Chinese character and sentence can present variations in meaning while lacking any grammatical aids or punctuation. The written language of the ancient Chinese was more suited for expressing philosophical ideas. Therefore, chapter by chapter this translation was born out of a slow and laborious process. Fortunately, I had at my disposal over twenty different interpretations and commentaries on the *Neijing* in Chinese. I was also able frequently to consult my father, himself a Chinese physician, and several *Neijing* scholars in China. Furthermore, I was assisted by able students and friends, who untiringly transcribed and helped polish the book into its present form.

This translation, however, was never meant to be a scholarly edition. For that purpose I am certain that other improvements can be made by expert sinologists. Instead, I have approached this from a clinician's point of view, all the while keeping in mind the criteria of students of traditional Chinese medicine and philosophy as well as those of interested laypersons.

I have taken much liberty in my humble attempt to convey the contents of the *Neijing*, such as eliminating the footnotes and instead incorporating them into the body of the translation. For instance, a direct translation of a sentence in chapter 3 would read: "Heaven gives birth to the five phases and the three qi." The more extended translation I have made appears in this book as: "The universal yin and yang transform into the five earthly transformative energies, also known as the five elemental phases, which consist of wood, fire, earth, metal, and water. These five elemental phases also correspond to the three yin and the three yang of the universe. These are the six atmospheric influences that govern the weather patterns that are reflected in changes in our planetary ecology."

It is my hope that by presenting a more accessible edition of this ancient classic to the modern reader, the world can benefit from its ideas and wisdom, and the way to health, happiness, and harmony can be attained by all people.

ACKNOWLEDGMENTS

I WOULD like to thank my father for pointing the way to the source of health and happiness. Respectful appreciation is also extended to Professors Peiran Qiu, Jianfu Jiang, Yingqiu Ren, Yaozhong Feng, and Jingcun Mung for their inspirations and generosity in imparting their insights on the *Neijing*. Particular thanks go to Dr. Pamela Speraw for encouraging and helping me initiate the project; Ms. Julie Chambers for typing and organizing the majority of the book; and Dr. Marc Chesler for editing and providing many invaluable feedbacks. I am indebted to my brother Dr. Daoshing Ni for helping me with chapters on the energetic phase. Special gratitude goes to Dr. Juen Wen for her dedicated efforts in assisting with the final manuscript while I was making a push for the completion of this book. Without everyone's support and understanding, this book might still be in my computer unfinished. I am grateful to my editor, Kendra Crossen, and publisher, Samuel Bercholz, of Shambhala Publications for their confidence and patience in this project.

PRONUNCIATION GUIDE

THE following table of the Pinyin phonetic alphabet shows pronunciations with approximate English equivalents. In parentheses are the corresponding letters in the Wade-Giles system.

a (a) as in *father*

b (p) as in *book*

c (ts', tz') like *ts* in *its*

ch (ch) as in *chin*, strongly aspirated

d (t) as in *duck*

e (e) as in *her*

f (f) as in *finger*

g (k) as in *get*

h (h) as in *her*, strongly aspirated

i (i) like the vowel sound in *eel* or the *i* in *sir*

j (ch) as in *jeer*

k (k') as in *kit*, strongly aspirated

l (l) as in *love*

m (m) as in *mine*

n (n) as in *not*

o (o) like the vowel sound in *law*

p (p') as in *pen*, strongly aspirated

q (ch') like the *ch* in *cheese*

r (j) as in *ring* or like the *z* in *azure*

s (s, ss, sz) as in *sister*

sh (sh) as in *show*

t (t') as in *tough*, strongly aspirated

u (u) as in *too*; also in the French *tu*

w (w) semi-vowel in syllables beginning with *u* when not preceded by consonants, pronounced as in *want*

x (hs) like *sh* in *sheet*

y semi-vowel in syllables beginning with *i* or *u* when not preceded by consonants, pronounced as in *yes*

z (ts, tz) as in *zero*

zh (ch) like the first consonant in *jump*

ai like *ie* in *pie*

ao like *ow* in *cow*

ei like *ay* in *day*

ie like *ie* in *experience*

ou like *oe* in *toe*

THE YELLOW EMPEROR'S
CLASSIC OF MEDICINE

CHAPTER 1

—

THE UNIVERSAL TRUTH

—

I N ancient times the Yellow Emperor, Huang Di, was known to have
been a child prodigy. As he grew he showed himself to be sincere, wise,
honest, and compassionate. He became very learned and developed keen
powers for observing nature. His people recognized him as a natural leader
and chose him as their emperor.

During his reign, Huang Di discoursed on medicine, health, lifestyle,
nutrition, and Taoist cosmology with his ministers Qi Bo, Lei Gong, and
others. Their first discussion began with Huang Di inquiring, "I've heard
that in the days of old everyone lived one hundred years without showing
the usual signs of aging. In our time, however, people age prematurely,
living only fifty years. Is this due to a change in the environment, or is it
because people have lost the correct way of life?"

Qi Bo replied, "In the past, people practiced the Tao, the Way of Life.
They understood the principle of balance, of yin and yang, as represented
by the transformation of the energies of the universe. Thus, they formu-
lated practices such as Dao-in, an exercise combining stretching, massaging,
and breathing to promote energy flow, and meditation to help maintain
and harmonize themselves with the universe. They ate a balanced diet at
regular times, arose and retired at regular hours, avoided overstressing their
bodies and minds, and refrained from overindulgence of all kinds. They
maintained well-being of body and mind; thus, it is not surprising that they
lived over one hundred years.

"These days, people have changed their way of life. They drink wine
as though it were water, indulge excessively in destructive activities, drain
their jing—the body's essence that is stored in the kidneys—and deplete
their qi. They do not know the secret of conserving their energy and vitality. Seeking emotional excitement and momentary pleasures, people disregard the natural rhythm and order of the universe. They fail to regulate
their lifestyle and diet, and sleep improperly. So it is not surprising that they
look old at fifty and die soon after.

"The accomplished ones of ancient times advised people to guard themselves against zei feng, disease-causing factors. On the mental level, one should remain calm and avoid excessive desires and fantasies, recognizing and maintaining the natural purity and clarity of the mind. When internal energies are able to circulate smoothly and freely, and the energy of the mind is not scattered, but is focused and concentrated, illness and disease can be avoided.

"Previously, people led a calm and honest existence, detached from undue desire and ambition; they lived with an untainted conscience and without fear. They were active, but never depleted themselves. Because they lived simply, these individuals knew contentment, as reflected in their diet of basic but nourishing foods and attire that was appropriate to the season but never luxurious. Since they were happy with their position in life, they did not feel jealousy or greed. They had compassion for others and were helpful and honest, free from destructive habits. They remained unshakable and unswayed by temptations, and they were able to stay centered even when adversity arose. They treated others justly, regardless of their level of intelligence or social position."

Huang Di asked, "When one grows old, one cannot bear children. Is this due to heredity or to the loss of one's procreative energy?"

Qi Bo answered, "In general, the reproductive physiology of woman is such that at seven years of age her kidney energy becomes full, her permanent teeth come in, and her hair grows long. At fourteen years the tian kui, or fertility essence, matures, the ren/conception and chong/vital channels responsible for conception open, menstruation begins, and conception is possible. At twenty-one years the kidney energy is strong and healthy, the wisdom teeth appear, and the body is vital and flourishing. At twenty-eight years the bones and tendons are well developed and the hair and secondary sex characteristics are complete. This is the height of female development. At thirty-five years the yangming/stomach and large intestine channels that govern the major facial muscles begin to deplete, the muscles begin to atrophy, facial wrinkles appear, and the hair begins to thin. At forty-two all three yang channels—taiyang, shaoyang, and yangming—are exhausted, the entire face is wrinkled, and the hair begins to turn gray. At forty-nine years the ren and chong channels are completely empty, and the tien kui has dried up. Hence, the flow of the menses ceases and the woman is no longer able to conceive.

"In the male, at eight years of age the kidney energy becomes full, the permanent teeth appear, and the hair becomes long. At sixteen years of age the kidney energy is ample, the tien kui is mature, and the jing is ripe, so procreation is possible. At twenty-four years the kidney qi is abundant, the bones and tendons grow strong, and the wisdom teeth come in. At the thirty-second year the body is at the peak of strength, and functions of the male are at their height. By forty the kidney qi begins to wane, teeth become loose, and the hair starts to fall. At forty-eight the yang energy of the head begins to deplete, the face becomes sallow, the hair grays, and the teeth deteriorate. By fifty-six years the liver energy weakens, causing the tendons to stiffen. At sixty-four the tian kui dries up and the jing is drained, resulting in kidney exhaustion, fatigue, and weakness. When the energy of all the organs is full, the excess energy stored in the kidney is excreted for the purpose of conception. But now, the organs have aged and their energies have become depleted, the bones and tendons have become frail and stiff, and movements are hampered. The kidney reservoir becomes empty, marking the end of the power of conception."

Huang Di remarked, "I notice, however, that some people, even though they are quite elderly, can still conceive."

Qi Bo replied, "This is because these individuals inherited an unusual abundance of jing and also realized how to lead their lives properly and protect their vitality. At sixty-four and forty-nine, for males and females respectively, these individuals still have excess kidney energy as well as qi and blood, so they still have the capacity to procreate. However, men past the age of sixty-four and women past forty-nine have normally lost this ability."

Huang Di asked, "If a wise one who follows the Tao is over one hundred years of age, can he or she still retain the ability to procreate?"

Qi Bo answered, "Yes, it is possible. If one knows how to live a correct way of life, conserve one's energy, and follow the Tao, yes, it is possible. One could procreate at the age of one hundred years."

Huang Di inquired, "I've heard of people in ancient times, spoken of as the immortals, who knew the secrets of the universe and held yin and yang, the world, in the palms of their hands. They extracted essence from nature and practiced various disciplines such as Dao-in and Qi Gong, and breathing and visualization exercises, to integrate the body, mind, and spirit. They remained undisturbed and thus attained extraordinary levels of accomplishment. Can you tell me about them?"

Qi Bo responded, "The immortals kept their mental energies focused and refined, and harmonized their bodies with the environment. Thus, they did not show conventional signs of aging and were able to live beyond biological limitations.

"Not so long ago there were people known as achieved beings who had true virtue, understood the way of life, and were able to adapt to and harmonize with the universe and the seasons. They too were able to keep their mental energy through proper concentration.

"These achieved beings did not live like ordinary humans, who tended to abuse themselves. They were able to travel freely to different times and places since they were not governed by conventional views of time and space. Their sense perceptions were supernormal, going far beyond the sight and hearing of ordinary humans. They were also able to preserve their life spans and live in full health, much as the immortals did.

"There was a third type of person, known as the sage. The sages lived peacefully under heaven on earth, following the rhythms of the planet and the universe. They adapted to society without being swayed by cultural trends. They were free from emotional extremes and lived a balanced, contented existence. Their outward appearance, behavior, and thinking did not reflect the conflicting norms of society. The sages appeared busy but were never depleted. Internally they did not overburden themselves. They abided in calmness, recognizing the empty nature of phenomenological existence. The sages lived over one hundred years because they did not scatter and disperse their energies.

"A fourth type were natural people who followed the Tao and were called naturalists. They lived in accordance with the rhythmic patterns of the seasons: heaven and earth, moon, sun, and stars. They aspired to follow the ways of ancient times, choosing not to lead excessive lifestyles. They, too, lived plainly and enjoyed long life."

CHAPTER 2

—

THE ART OF LIFE THROUGH THE FOUR SEASONS

—

HUANG DI said, "The three months of the spring season bring about the revitalization of all things in nature. It is the time of birth. This is when heaven and earth are reborn. During this season it is advisable to retire early. Arise early also and go walking in order to absorb the fresh, invigorating energy. Since this is the season in which the universal energy begins anew and rejuvenates, one should attempt to correspond to it directly by being open and unsuppressed, both physically and emotionally.

"On the physical level it is good to exercise more frequently and wear loose-fitting clothing. This is the time to do stretching exercises to loosen up the tendons and muscles. Emotionally, it is good to develop equanimity. This is because spring is the season of the liver, and indulgence in anger, frustration, depression, sadness, or any excess emotion can injure the liver. Furthermore, violating the natural order of spring will cause cold disease, illness inflicted by atmospheric cold, during summer.

"In the three months of summer there is an abundance of sunshine and rain. The heavenly energy descends, and the earthly energy rises. When these energies merge there is intercourse between heaven and earth. As a result plants mature and animals, flowers, and fruit appear abundantly.

"One may retire somewhat later at this time of year, while still arising early. One should refrain from anger and stay physically active, to prevent the pores from closing and the qi from stagnating. One should not overindulge in sex, although one can indulge a bit more than in other seasons. Emotionally, it is important to be happy and easygoing and not hold grudges, so that the energy can flow freely and communicate between the external and the internal. In this way illness may be averted in the fall. The season of fire and heart also encompasses late summer, which corresponds to the earth element. Problems in the summer will cause injury to the heart and will manifest in the autumn.

"In the three months of autumn all things in nature reach their full maturity. The grains ripen and harvesting occurs. The heavenly energy cools, as does the weather. The wind begins to stir. This is the changing or privoting point when the yang, or active, phase turns into its opposite, the yin, or passive, phase. One should retire with the sunset and arise with the dawn. Just as the weather in autumn turns harsh, so does the emotional climate. It is therefore important to remain calm and peaceful, refraining from depression so that one can make the transition to winter smoothly. This is the time to gather one's spirit and energy, be more focused, and not allow desires to run wild. One must keep the lung energy full, clean, and quiet. This means practicing breathing exercises to enhance lung qi. Also, one should refrain from both smoking and grief, the emotion of the lung. This will prevent kidney or digestive problems in the winter. If this natural order is violated, damage will occur to the lungs, resulting in diarrhea with undigested food in winter. This compromises the body's ability to store in winter.

"During the winter months all things in nature wither, hide, return home, and enter a resting period, just as lakes and rivers freeze and snow falls. This is a time when yin dominates yang. Therefore one should refrain from overusing the yang energy. Retire early and get up with the sunrise, which is later in winter. Desires and mental activity should be kept quiet and subdued. Sexual desires especially should be contained, as if keeping a happy secret. Stay warm, avoid the cold, and keep the pores closed. Avoid sweating. The philosophy of the winter season is one of conservation and storage. Without such practice the result will be injury to the kidney energy. This will cause wei jue, consisting of weakness, atrophy of muscles, and coldness in spring, manifesting as paralysis, wei/flaccid syndrome, arthritis, or degeneration of the bones and tendons. This is because the body has lost its ability to open and move in the spring.

"So the full cycle can be seen. Spring is the beginning of things, when the energy should be kept open and fluid; summer opens up further into an exchange or communication between internal and external energies; in the fall it is important to conserve; finally, the winter is dominated by the storage of energy."

Huang Di continued, "The heavenly energy is bright and clear, continually circulates, and has great virtue. This is because it does not radiate its brilliance, for if it did proclaim itself, neither the sun nor the moon would be visible. People should follow the virtuous way of heaven, not exposing their true energy. In this way they will not lose it or be subject to attacks of evil energies, which produce illness in the body. If the body is attacked by evil energy, its own energy will become stuck, just as when the clouds cover the sky, obscuring the sun and moon and causing darkness.

"The heavenly energy naturally circulates and communicates with the earth's energy; the heavenly energy descends and the earthly energy ascends. When this intercourse takes place and these energies merge, the result is a balance of sunshine and rain, wind and frost, and the four seasons. If the heavenly energy becomes stuck, sunshine and rain cannot come forth. Without them, all living things cease to be nourished and lose their vitality, and imbalance manifests as storms and hurricanes; severe and harsh weather disrupts the natural order, causing chaos and destruction.

"In the past the sages were able to observe the signs and adapt themselves to these natural phenomena so that they were unaffected by exogenous influences, or "evil wind," and were able to live long lives. If one does not follow the play of the elemental energies according to the seasons, the liver energy will stagnate, resulting in illness in spring. In summer, the heart energy becomes empty and the yang energy is exhausted. During the autumn there will be congestion of the lung energy. In winter the kidney will be drained of jing.

"The transformation of yin and yang in the four seasons is the basis of the growth and the destruction of life. The sages were able to cultivate the yang energy in spring and summer and conserve the yin energy in autumn and winter. By following the universal order, growth can occur naturally. If this natural order is disregarded, the root of one's life will be damaged and one's true energy will wane.

"Therefore, the change of yin and yang through the four seasons is the root of life, growth, reproduction, aging, and destruction. By respecting this natural law it is possible to be free from illness. The sages have followed this, and the foolish people have not.

"In the old days the sages treated disease by preventing illness before it began, just as a good government or emperor was able to take the necessary steps to avert war. Treating an illness after it has begun is like suppressing revolt after it has broken out. If someone digs a well when thirsty, or forges weapons after becoming engaged in battle, one cannot help but ask: Are not these actions too late?"

CHAPTER 3

—

THE UNION OF HEAVEN
AND HUMAN BEINGS

—

HUANG DI said, "From ancient times it has been recognized that there is an intimate relationship between the activity and life of human beings and their natural environment. The root of all life is yin and yang; this includes everything in the universe, with heaven above and earth below, within the four directions and the nine continents. In the human body there are the nine orifices of ears, eyes, nostrils, mouth, anus, and urethra; the five zang organs of kidneys, liver, heart, spleen, and lungs; and the twelve joints of elbows, wrists, knees, ankles, shoulders, and hips, which are all connected with the qi of the universe. The universal yin and yang transform into the five earthly transformative energies, also known as the five elemental phases that consist of wood, fire, earth, metal, and water.

"These five elemental phases also correspond to the three yin and the three yang of the universe. These are the six atmospheric influences that govern the weather patterns that reflect in changes in our planetary ecology. If people violate or disrupt this natural order, then pathogenic forces will have an opportunity to cause damage to the body.

"The yang qi of the body is like the sun. If the sun loses its brilliance or illuminating effect, all things on earth become inactive. The sun is the ultimate yang. This heavenly energy of the sun, yang qi, surrounds the earth. Correspondingly, in the body this means that the yang qi circulates around the center or core and has the function of protecting the body."

Huang Di continued, "Living in a cold climate, one must take extra care with one's activities. Just as people indoors are protected from harsh weather, the yang qi acts as the walls in a house to protect the body. It is important to be orderly and not allow any openings; pathogenic energy cannot invade if the castle doors are closed.

"During the winter, if one lives improperly, giving in to impulsive

desires and emotions such as anger and irritability, the spirit becomes restless, causing the yang qi to disperse at the surface. At this point the yang qi
can no longer control the orifices and pores of the body. The result will be
an outpouring of the qi and subsequent vulnerability to invasions.

"In the summer, if too much sweating occurs in the heat, the qi will
escape, the breath will become coarse and rapid, and one will feel irritable.
These are the symptoms of heat attacking the exterior.

"If summer heat attacks and enters the interior, it will affect the mind
and spirit, causing delirium, muttering, and fever. In order to relieve these
symptoms, the pores must be opened to release the heat.

"When damp invades the body, the head will feel heavy and distended, as if tightly bandaged. The large muscles and tendons will contract,
and the small muscles and tendons will become flaccid, resulting in loss of
mobility, spasms, and atrophy.

"A blockage of qi due to deficiency will cause the extremities to become swollen and movement to be impaired. This is indicative of the
exhaustion of the yang qi.

"When one is overworked and overstressed, the yang will overheat,
eventually depleting the yin and jing/essence. If this continues into the
summer, the body fluids and yin will be dehydrated. This is known as the
jian jue syndrome, syncope caused by the consumption of yin fluids, with
symptoms of blurred vision, deafness, and ear congestion. Further, if one
indulges in extreme anger, it will force the energy to flow recklessly, obstructing blood flow in the head, resulting in syncope. When this type of
congealing takes place, it is known as bo jue, syncope due to a battle between qi and blood.

"When the tendons become damaged they lose their elasticity and
contractibility; thus mobility becomes impaired. Sweating on only one side
of the body is a warning sign of pian ku, hemiplegia. If the pores are open
and dampness invades, this can cause zuo fei—rash, dermatitis, and furun-
cle. Consuming large amounts of rich, greasy food can induce ding chuang,
larger lesions with pus.

"After heavy exertion and sweating, wind and cold can invade the
skin, causing zha, or red spots on the nose. If this wind and cold are allowed
to accumulate over a long period, there will be zuo chuang, lesions on the
buttocks and in the rectal area, with ulcerations and boils.

"The yang qi transforms the jing/essence to nourish the shen/spirit
and harmonizes with the ying qi to sustain the tendons. Should the skin

pores lose their regulating function, the pathogenic cold can enter, and the yang qi becomes obstructed or damaged. Tendons will then lose their source of nourishment, and the body will become stiff and movement difficult and painful.

"If the pathogenic cold penetrates deeper to the blood level, obstruction of blood and bruising will be seen and will lead to lou, perforated scrofula of the neck. At the muscle level, lesions and wounds will not close or heal properly.

"When cold invades through the shu/transport points of the acupuncture meridians and continues to move through the circulation into the organs, it will manifest as fear, fright, or startling nightmares.

"The ying/nutritive qi usually flows in the channels, but if pathogenic cold is present and the ying qi is blocked in the muscles, yong zhong, suppurative swelling with cysts and pus conditions will manifest. If a weak person sweats excessively, wind and cold can obstruct the pores, and fluid will accumulate in the muscle level. The shu/transport points can become blocked, causing feng nui, wind malaria with alternating chills and fever, headache, and irritability.

"Pathogenic wind is the root of all evil. However, if one is centered and the emotions are clear and calm, energy is abundant and resistance is strong; even when confronted with the force of the most powerful, vicious wind, one will not be invaded. When it remains in the body for a long time, the pathogenic factor will transform, internalize, and stagnate to the point where the flow of qi is impaired, from top to bottom, side to side, or between yin and yang. Even the most accomplished doctor finds it difficult to remedy this condition. When the yang qi is stuck, it is necessary to purge with herbs and sedate promptly with acupuncture; otherwise, death may result. A mediocre doctor may not recognize the severe consequences of yang qi that has become stuck.

"The yang qi moves like the sun. As the sun begins to rise at dawn, the yang qi begins to move to the outer body, and the pores open. The peak of the yang qi is at noon, and when the yang qi is most active it is advisable to relax and stay quiet so that the yang qi does not escape. As the sun sets, the yang qi moves inward and the pores begin to close. At this time it is harmful to engage in strenuous physical activity or expose oneself to cold, damp, mist, or fog. If one violates the natural order of the yang qi as it rises, peaks, and sets, the body will gradually be weakened by pathogenic factors and be subject to disease and degeneration."

Qi Bo added to the discussion: "Yin is the essence of the organs and the fountain of the qi. Yang protects the exterior of the body against pathogens and makes the muscles function. When the yin fails to contain the yang, the flow in the channels will become rapid, causing the yang qi to become excessive and reckless. If the yang qi is deficient and unable to counterbalance the yin, communication between the internal organs will be disrupted, and the nine orifices will cease to function. The sages, who understood the principles of yin and yang, were able to let their bodies perform all functions harmoniously. When yin and yang are balanced, the five zang organs function appropriately together; the tendons, ligaments, vessels, channels, and collaterals all flow smoothly; the muscles, bones, and marrow are abundant and strong, qi and blood follow the right path, internal and external are synergetic, vision is clear, and hearing is acute. Thus the zhen/true qi becomes unshakable, and pathogens cannot invade.

"When the evil wind invades the body, it gradually turns to heat and consumes the body's qi, jing/essence, and blood. When the blood becomes depleted, the liver is not nourished and it malfunctions.

"If one overeats, the muscles and blood vessels of the stomach and intestines overexpand and suffer from food retention. This leads to dysentery and hemorrhoids. Overindulgence in alcohol causes the energy to rise to the head. If intercourse is attempted, the energy will not be in the right place and the kidney qi will be drained, causing damage and degeneration of the low back. When qi is not in the kidneys during sex, the body will draw qi from the bones and marrow.

"The key to mastering health is to regulate the yin and the yang of the body. If the yin and yang balance is disrupted, it is like going through a year with spring but no winter, or winter but no summer. When the yang is excessive and cannot contain itself, the yin will become consumed. Only when the yin remains calm and harmonious will the yang qi be contained and not be overly expansive, the spirit normal, and the mind clear. If the yin and the yang separate, the jing/essence and the shen/spirit will also leave each other.

"When one is attacked by wind and exposed to fog, a condition of heat and cold will ensue. If during spring one is affected by wind that is not expelled, it will attack the spleen, causing diarrhea, indigestion, and food retention.

"If during the summer one is invaded by summer heat, malaria may occur in the autumn. During the autumn, if one is affected by dampness and the damp accumulates in the lung, it will cause wei jue, cold limbs with flaccidity, cough, and emaciation of the body and limbs. Cold invading in winter will incubate and manifest as febrile disease in spring, because everything rises at that time of year. The seasonal changes can cause damage to the organs if one is not careful and strong.

"The source and preservation of the yin come from the five flavors of food in the diet, but improper use of the five flavors may also injure the five zang organs. Too much sour taste may cause overactivity of the liver and underactivity of the spleen. Too much salty taste can weaken the bones and cause contracture and atrophy of the muscles, as well as stagnate the heart qi. Too much sweet taste can disturb the heart qi, causing it to become restless and congested, as well as cause imbalance of kidney energy, which turns the face black. Too much bitter taste disrupts the spleen's ability to transform and transport food, and causes the stomach to digest ineffectively and become distended. The muscles and tendons may become scattered.

"Therefore, one should be mindful of what one consumes to insure proper growth, reproduction, and development of bones, tendons, ligaments, channels, and collaterals. This will help generate the smooth flow of qi and blood, enabling one to live to a ripe age."

CHAPTER 4

—

THE TRUTH FROM
THE GOLDEN CHAMBER

—

HUANG DI said, "In nature there are eight types of wind, and within the body's channels and collaterals there are five types of wind. What do they mean?"

Qi Bo answered, "The eight types of wind that occur in nature are abnormal and pathogenic winds, which cause disease. These can affect the body's channels and collaterals, producing five types of internal wind that damage their corresponding organs. These internal winds are liver wind, heart wind, lung wind, kidney wind, and spleen wind. They are caused by abnormal changes in the four seasons. For example, spring overacts on late summer, late summer overacts on winter, winter overacts on summer, summer overacts on autumn, and autumn overacts on spring. This represents the control cycle of five element interactions in nature.

"In terms of five element correspondences, the spring element is related to wood, summer correlates to fire, late summer is earth, autumn is metal, and winter is water. The corresponding organs of these elements are: wood/liver, fire/heart, earth/spleen, metal/lungs, water/kidneys. During the spring the weather and environmental conditions can affect the liver, while in summer the heart can be affected, and so forth.

"If spring overacts on late summer, the weather is abnormal, with spring weather then occurring in late summer. The body's reaction to this is excessive liver/wood energy that overacts on the spleen/earth. When the late summer overacts on winter to create the weather of late summer in winter, the spleen/earth will overact on the kidneys/water. If winter overacts on summer, there will be cold spells of winter during summer. The kidneys/water will then become excessive and put out the heart/fire. When summer overacts on autumn and there is summer weather in autumn, this will cause heart/fire to flare up and attack the lungs/metal.

When autumn overacts on spring, the spring will be very dry and windy, as in autumn. Thus the lungs/metal will become overactive and impede the function of the liver/wood.

"When the seasons do not follow their natural cycle—spring, summer, late summer, autumn, winter—with the appropriate weather patterns and energetic transformations, colds, flu, and various illnesses will result.

"In the spring the wind comes from the east. Illness then occurs in the liver channel and rises to the head, causing bleeding from the nose. Acupuncture points on the neck and gallbladder channel should be used for treatment. In the summer the wind arises in the southern direction and affects the heart. To treat this, points on the chest and ribs should be employed. The westerly wind of autumn will affect the lungs, manifesting in malaria with alternating chills and fever. Points on the shoulders and upper back are useful in treatment. The northern winds of winter will affect the kidneys and limbs, manifesting in bi syndrome, a condition of obstruction of qi and blood, which typically results in stiffness, immobility, and pain in the joints. Acupuncture points on the lower back and buttocks can be used to treat this condition. Late summer is the hinge between hot and cold seasons, uniting the yin and the yang. This transitional period will mainly affect the spleen, causing internal colds with diarrhea. Points in the midback can be used.

"To preserve health in winter, one should not exercise excessively, since this will cause the yang qi to come to the surface instead of naturally going inward. Then the yang qi will become stuck in the head area, leading to nosebleeds and problems of the head and neck when spring arrives. In the summer there may be chest and rib problems; in the late summer, internal cold with diarrhea; in the winter, indigestion, bi or arthralgia syndrome, and excessive sweating. If the yang qi is in its proper place, all these seasonal problems can be averted.

"The sage knows that the jing/essence is the most precious substance in the body. Like the root of a tree, it should be protected and hidden from 'thieves' so that in spring there will not be febrile disease. Also, if one does not sweat and cool off during the hot summer, malarial types of disorders will develop in the ensuing autumn. It is therefore essential to protect the jing/essence by observing and adapting to the seasonal rhythms.

"It is said there is yin within yang and yang within yin. The day is considered yang, while the night is yin. This is further differentiated as follows: sunrise to noon is yang within yang; noon to sunset is yin within yang; twilight to midnight is yin within yin; midnight to sunrise is yang within yin.

"The kind of classification can also be applied to the human body. The outside of the body is considered yang, while the inside is yin. The back is yang and the front is yin. The upper half of the body is yang, while the lower half is yin. In terms of the zang fu organs, the heart, liver, spleen, lungs, and kidneys are the zang organs, since they are yin in nature and their function is transformation and storage. The gallbladder, stomach, large intestine, small intestine, bladder, and sanjiao (the three viscera cavities responsible for fluid metabolism) are the six fu or hollow organs, and they are considered yang. Their function is reception and passage. The concept of yin within yin and yang within yang can be understood by when and where disease occurs. For instance, an illness of winter occurs in the yin part of the body, a summer illness in the yang part; a spring disease in the yin part and an autumn disease in the yang part. One will then treat with acupuncture points according to the location of the disease.

"To further categorize, the chest area is considered yang, while the abdomen is yin. The heart and lungs are therefore yang types of zang organs. The heart is yang within yang, while the lung is yin within yang. Below the diaphragm in the abdomen we have the yin zang organs: liver, spleen, and kidneys. The kidneys are yin within yin, the liver yang within yin, and the spleen is utmost yin within yin. This classification helps one to understand the relative relationships between the organs and the body as a whole in terms of location, function, and nature of each organ."

Huang Di inquired, "The five zang organs correspond to the seasons. Do they each have other correspondences, and how do these affect the energy flow?"

Qi Bo replied, "In the east we have the green color, an energy which corresponds to the liver. The liver energy opens to the eyes. Illness may manifest as startling, fright, or shock. The natural elements related to this are grass and trees, the flavor is sour, the animal is the chicken, the grain is wheat, the planet is Sui/Jupiter, the number is 5, the smell is urine, the season is spring, the energy is ascending, and the area affected is the head. The liver controls the tendons."

Qi Bo then listed the five elements and their corresponding natures. [See table on page 16.]

Qi Bo added, "An effective doctor and diagnostician is able to observe the changes and transformations of the five zang and the six fu organs. He

	WOOD	FIRE	EARTH	METAL	WATER
DIRECTION	EAST	SOUTH	CENTRAL	WEST	NORTH
SEASON	SPRING	SUMMER	LATE SUMMER	AUTUMN	WINTER
WEATHER	WIND	HEAT	DAMP	DRYNESS	COLD
PLANET	SUI/JUPITER	RONGHUO/MARS	ZHENG/SATURN	TAI BAI/VENUS	CHEN/MERCURY
NUMEROLOGY	$3 + 5 = 8$	$2 + 5 = 7$	5	$4 + 5 = 9$	$1 + 5 = 6$
NATURAL ELEMENT	TREES/GRASS	FIRE	DIRT/EARTH	METAL	WATER
ANIMAL	CHICKEN	GOAT	COW	HORSE	PIG
CEREAL/GRAIN	WHEAT	CORN	RYE	RICE	BEAN
MUSICAL NOTE	JIAO/LUTE	ZHI/PIPE ORGAN	GONG/DRUM	SHANG/RESONANT	YU/STRINGED
COLOR	GREEN	RED	YELLOW	WHITE	BLACK
FLAVOR	SOUR	BITTER	SWEET	PUNGENT	SALTY
SMELL	URINE	SCORCHED	FRAGRANT	FISHY	ROTTEN
ZANG ORGAN	LIVER	HEART	SPLEEN	LUNG	KIDNEY
ORIFICE	EYES	EAR	MOUTH	NOSE	ANUS/URETHRA
BODY PART	TENDON/LIGAMENTS	VESSELS	MUSCLES/FLESH	SKIN/HAIR	BONES/MARROW
SOUND	SHOUT	LAUGHTER	SINGING/MELODIC	CRYING/WEEPING	MOANING
EMOTION	ANGER	JOY	DISTRESS/WORRY	GRIEF/SADNESS	FEAR
PATHOLOGICAL ACTIONS	CLENCH FIST/SPASMS	ANXIOUS LOOK	SPITTING	COUGH	SHIVERING
LOCATION	NECK/HEAD	CHEST/RIBS	MIDBACK	SHOULDER/UPPER BACK	LOW BACK HIPS/LIMBS
SPIRIT	HUN/SOUL	SHEN/SPIRIT	YI/LOGIC	PO/COURAGE	ZHI/WILL

knows the corresponding external factors and transformational energies, the yin and yang, the six atmospheric influences of heat, cold, wind, damp, dryness, and summer heat. The accomplished doctor is able to follow illnesses both on the surface and internally, and see the direction and progression of a disease. All these correspondences will aid the doctor in effectively diagnosing and dispensing treatment to the patient. This is the Tao.

"The Tao is precious and is not to be passed on unless a student is sincere and compassionate toward human suffering. Only in this way can the great tradition remain pure and virtuous."

CHAPTER 5

—

THE MANIFESTATION OF YIN AND YANG FROM THE MACROCOSM TO THE MICROCOSM

—

H UANG DI said, "The law of yin and yang is the natural order of the universe, the foundation of all things, mother of all changes, the root of life and death. In healing, one must grasp the root of the disharmony, which is always subject to the law of yin and yang.

"In the universe, the pure yang qi ascends to converge and form heaven, while the turbid yin qi descends and condenses to form the earth. Yin is passive and quiet, while the nature of yang is active and noisy. Yang is responsible for expanding and yin is responsible for contracting, becoming astringent, and consolidating. Yang is the energy, the vital force, the potential, while yin is the substance, the foundation, the mother that gives rise to all this potential.

"Extreme heat or extreme cold will transform into its opposite. For example, on a hot day the heat will rise, causing condensation and eventually rain and therefore cold.

"Coldness produces turbid yin, heat produces the clear yang. If the clear yang qi descends instead of rising, problems such as diarrhea occur in the body. If the turbid yin qi becomes stuck at the top and fails to descend, there will be fullness and distension in the head. These conditions are imbalances of yin and yang.

"In nature, the clear yang forms heaven and the turbid yin qi descends to form earth. The earthly qi evaporates to become the clouds, and when the clouds meet with the heavenly qi, rain is produced. Similarly, in the body, pure yang qi reaches the sensory orifices, allowing one to see, hear, smell, taste, feel, and decipher all information so that the shen/spirit can remain clear and centered. The turbid yin qi descends to the lower orifices.

The clear yang qi disperses over the surface of the body; the turbid yin qi flows and nourishes the five zang organs. The pure yang qi expands and strengthens the four extremities, and the turbid yin qi fills the six fu organs.

"The elements of fire and water are categorized into yang and yin, the fire being yang and the water being yin. The functional aspect of the body is yang and the nutritive or substantive aspect is yin. While food can be used to strengthen and nourish the body, the body's ability to transform it is dependent on qi. The functional part of the qi is derived from the jing/essence. Food is refined into jing/essence, which supports the qi, and the qi is required for both transformation and bodily functions. For this reason, when the diet is improper, the body may be injured, or if activities are excessive, the jing/essence qi can be exhausted.

"Taste is a yin quality and has a descending nature, while qi is yang and rises to the upper orifices. Heavy tastes are pure yin, light tastes are considered yang within yin. The heavier qi is pure yang in nature while the lighter qi is yin within yang.

"When taste or food is heavy and turbid, it may cause diarrhea, but the lighter, refined taste is able to circulate throughout the meridians. It is therefore advisable to eat simple, bland foods rather than rich ones.

"The lighter qi is expansive and has a tendency to disperse out of the body through the pores and orifices. The heavier, more substantial qi can assist the yang to produce fire in the body. If there is an excess of the yang/fire, it can damage the body's yuan/source qi, so it is advisable to avoid creating excess fire in the body.

"A taste is related to its energetic properties. The pungent and sweet tastes that have dispersing qualities are considered yang, while the sour and bitter tastes that have purging and eliminating qualities are considered yin.

"The yin and yang in the body should be in balance with one another. If the yang qi dominates, the yin will be deprived, and vice versa. Excess yang will manifest as febrile disease, whereas excess yin will manifest as cold disease. When yang is extreme, however, it can turn into cold disease, and vice versa.

"Cold can injure the physical body, and heat can damage the qi or energetic aspect of the body. When there is injury to the physical body there will be swelling, but if the qi level is damaged, it can cause pain because of the qi blockage. In an injury that has two aspects, such as swelling (yin) and pain (yang), treatment may consist of pungent herbs to disperse swelling and cooling herbs to subdue the pain. If a patient complains of pain first and swelling afterward, this means the qi level was injured first. But if a patient complains of swelling first followed by pain, the trauma occurred at the physical level initially."

Huang Di continued: "When the pathogenic wind comes like a storm, it can cause shaking. If fire burns excessively, there will be redness and swelling; if dryness is present, there will be withering; excess cold can result in swelling; and extreme dampness will lead to urinary problems and diarrhea."

"In nature, we have the four seasons and the five energetic transformations of wood, fire, earth, metal, and water. Their changes and transformations produce cold, summer heat, dampness, dryness, and wind. The weather, in turn, affects every living creature in the natural world and forms the foundation for birth, growth, maturation, and death.

"In the human body there are the zang organs of the liver, heart, spleen, lung, and kidneys. The qi of the five zang organs forms the five spirits and gives rise to the five emotions. The spirit of the heart is known as the shen, which rules mental and creative functions. The spirit of the liver, the hun, rules the nervous system and gives rise to extrasensory perception. The spirit of the spleen, of yi, rules logic or reasoning power. The spirit of the lungs, or po, rules the animalistic instincts, physical strength and stamina. The spirit of the kidneys, the zhi, rules the will, drive, ambition, and survival instinct.

"Overindulgence in the five emotions—happiness, anger, sadness, worry or fear, and fright—can create imbalances. Emotions can injure the qi, while seasonal elements can attack the body. Sudden anger damages the yin qi; becoming easily excited or overjoyed will damage the yang qi. This causes the qi to rebel and rise up to the head, squeezing the shen out of the heart and allowing it to float away. Failing to regulate one's emotions can be likened to summer and winter failing to regulate each other, threatening life itself.

"If there is cold invasion in the winter, febrile disease will develop in the spring. An invasion by wind in the spring can result in digestive disturbances, food retention, and diarrhea in the summer. If there is an attack of summer heat during the summer, in the autumn there may be malaria. If dampness invades in the autumn, there will be coughing attacks in the winter."

Huang Di then asked, "I have heard that in ancient times, persons educated in medicine emphasized the physical body by differentiating the zang fu, understood the distribution and function of the channels and collaterals, and gave names to the points of qi, or acupuncture points. In the muscles and spaces between the muscles and the joints can be found the points that connect the meridians. The meridians are further coupled as yin/yang pairs, called liu he. Everything is distributed perfectly, corresponding to the yin and the yang and the four seasons in harmony with the universe. Is what the ancient ones said accurate?"

Qi Bo answered, "With the arrival of spring the weather warms the earth. All plants begin to sprout and put forth green leaves, so the color associated with spring is green. Since most fruits and trees are immature and unripe at this time, their taste is sour. This sour taste can strengthen the liver, and the liver can then nourish the tendons and tendomuscular channels. The wood element of the liver can produce the fire element of the heart; thus, it is said that the tendons produce the heart. Liver connects with the eyes through its channels, and thus it is said that the upper orifice of the liver is the eyes.

"During spring the subtlety and vastness of the universe, the intelligence and intuition of the human being, the ability of the earth to produce the ten thousand things, the natural movement of the wind, and the upward motion of all plants, collectively produce the movement of the tendons, the color green, the shouting of the voice, the spasms and convulsions, the eyes, the sour taste, and the angry emotions. These are all associated with the liver, since the liver is responsible for maintaining the patency of the flow of energy, and its nature is movement and expansion.

"Anger can injure the liver, but sadness can relieve anger. When wind invades with dampness, it can injure the tendons, although dryness may eliminate the dampness and wind. Excessive consumption of sour foods can make the tendons flaccid, but this can be neutralized by the pungent taste.

"In summer the weather is generally hot, and when there is extreme heat it produces fire, which can burn and char things, producing the bitter taste. Bitter-tasting substances can clear the heart. The heart governs the blood, the fire of the heart produces the earth, the heart opens to the tongue, and therefore subtle changes in the heart can be reflected in the tongue.

"The hot weather, the fire on the planet, the blood vessels, the color red, laughter, and joy are all related to the heart. The heart, or fire element, manifests emotionally as joy, but too much joy can cause a depletion of the heart qi. This can be counterbalanced by fear. Pathogenic qi can invade the heart via the pericardium, injuring heart qi. Cold and cooling herbs can be useful to counteract this condition. Consuming overly bitter foods can have a harmful effect on the heart qi, but salty foods can be used to balance the excess bitter.

"In the center we find dampness and humidity, which can nourish and lubricate the soil, preparing it to produce strong earth. During the season between summer and autumn, late summer, the fruits ripen and turn yellow. When they ripen they taste sweet and can nourish spleen qi. The spleen qi is then able to nourish the muscles and flesh. From the supple flesh and muscles the lungs are generated; these correspond to the metal element. The spleen opens to the mouth, and diseases of the spleen can enter through the mouth and will be reflected on the lips.

"On earth the weather correlation would be damp and humid conditions. The spleen manifests in the muscles and flesh; the color yellow is associated with the spleen, as is a singing, melodic voice. Pathologic conditions of turbidity indicate spleen imbalance. Melancholy and overworry will manifest. Excessive worry will deplete spleen qi, but anger can restrain this worry. Dampness can damage flesh and muscles, but wind can dry the damp. Too much sweet taste can injure the flesh by creating fat, but sour can neutralize the sweet.

"In the western direction the deserts are rich in metal ores; the dry desert sands are white, and this dryness affects the lungs, skin, hair, and pores of the body. The sound of crying and the emotion of sadness and grief are associated with the metal element. The pungent taste can ventilate the lungs and open the pores. Extreme grief can injure the lungs, but may be counteracted by the emotion of happiness. Intense heat can damage the skin, hair, and lungs. In this case, coldness is required to control the pathogen. Excessive consumption of the pungent taste may injure the pores and skin, but this can be counteracted by the bitter taste.

"In the northern direction there are vast snow-covered mountain ranges, and beyond, dark and cold seas whose ocean waters provide the salty taste. All of these conditions are connected with the kidney energy and enable it to develop strong, healthy bones and marrow. The kidneys are associated with the ears, the color black, fear and fright, and the sound of moaning. While fear and fright will damage the kidneys, understanding, logic, and rational thinking will enable one to defeat the fright. Coldness will slow down and stagnate the blood, but dryness will temper this harshness. Excesses of salty flavor can harm the blood, but the sweet flavor will neutralize it.

"Heaven and earth, the masculine and feminine principles, the qi and the blood, all reflect the interplay of yin and yang. Water has the property of coldness, fire the property of heat. The interdependence of yin and yang is reflected in all things in the universe and cannot be separated."

Huang Di asked, "How would you apply the principle of yin and yang to the art of healing?"

Qi Bo replied, "If the yang qi is in excess, the body will have fever, difficult, rapid breathing, tremors and shaking, dry throat and mouth, irritability, and abdominal distension. These signs are the precursors of death. When an excess of yang qi occurs in the winter, it is not as dangerous as in the summer, when environmental heat will rapidly worsen it.

"If the yin qi becomes excessive, the body will feel cold, there will be clammy sweating, shivering, and convulsive spasms of the hands and feet. If the extremities are in spasm and the abdomen is swollen and distended, this will warn of death. During the summer it will be possible to recover, but in the winter it will be fatal. So we can see the manifestation of yin and yang in the process of disease."

Then Huang Di inquired, "What are the methods to balance yin and yang?"

Qi Bo answered, "If one understands the methods or Tao of maintaining health and the causes of depletion, then one can readily master the balance of yin and yang and stay healthy. Normally, by the age of forty, people have exhausted fifty percent of their yin qi, and their vitality is weakened. At age fifty the body is heavy, the vision and the hearing deteriorated; by age sixty the yin qi is further diminished, the kidneys drained; the sensory organs and the nine orifices, including the excretory organs, have all become functionally impaired. Conditions will manifest such as prostatitis, vision loss, deficiency in the lower jiao (viscera cavity) and excess in the upper jiao, tearing, and nasal drainage problems.

"Thus, the body of one who understands the Tao will remain strong and healthy. The one who does not understand the Tao will age. One who is careless will often feel deficient, while one who knows will have an abundance of energy. Those who are knowledgeable have clear orifices, perceptions, hearing, vision, smell, and taste, and are light and strong. Even though their bodies are old, they can perform most of life's activities.

"Those who understand the principles of wholesome living tame their minds and prevent them from straying. They do not force anything upon themselves or others, are happy and content, tranquil and quiet, and can live indefinitely. These are the ancient methods of self-maintenance."

Qi Bo continued, "In the northwest direction the mountains are high and cold and are considered yin, while in the southwest the lowlands are hot and yang in nature. There is a correspondence between heaven and humankind. Just as there are inequalities in nature, such as hot and cold, high and low, so they also exist in people. In the body, the right ear is not as effective as the left, nor is the right eye as sharp as the left. However, the left hand and foot are not as coordinated as the right, in general."

Huang Di asked, "What does this mean?"

Qi Bo answered, "The east is the yang direction. The essence of yang circulates from the left, rises in the left, and the upper left side is full while the bottom left is deficient. The western direction is considered yin, and the essence of yin descends down the right side. Therefore, the lower right is full and the upper right is deficient. This is why we say the right eye and ear are not as strong as the left, and the left hand and foot are not as strong as the right.

"It is important to understand that the pathogen always attacks where there is deficiency. In human beings, the right upper and left lower are both deficient and therefore vulnerable to pathogenic attacks. These are natural flaws that have been created.

"Heaven produces qi. Earth gives rise to form. Heaven regulates the four seasons. On earth the transformations of the five elements represent the interplay of yin and yang. Yang rises to produce heaven, while the turbid yin descends to form the earth. This movement helps create the rhythm of the seasons and the weather changes, enabling earthly things to manifest in the rhythm of birth in spring, growth in summer, consolidation in autumn, and storage in winter. Possessing this knowledge, people can coordinate their activities around these cycles and benefit by them, since human life is interconnected with its environment, heaven and earth.

"The heavenly qi travels through the lungs, and the earthly water and grains, or substantial qi, travels through the throat. The qi of the winds and trees connects with the liver, the thundering fire qi connects with the heart, the qi of the five grains from the earth connects with the spleen, and the rainwater qi connects to the kidneys. The movement and traveling of qi and blood in the six channels is like a river flowing; and the stomach and large intestine, which contain the fluids and food, are like the ocean. The nine orifices are like the spring where water gushes in and out. The yin and yang of the human body can thus be related to the phenomena of nature. The sweat from excess yang pours out like rain, the active yang qi moves like rapid wind, the anger of people is like the raging of thunder. Rebellious qi that rushes upward is like the blazing of fire. Without understanding the metaphors present in nature and humans, one will not effectively avert or treat disease. In treatment, when one neglects to take the seasonal changes into consideration and fails to recognize the geography, the environment, the five elements and their transformations, one will miss the big picture and treatment will be unsuccessful. This is the importance of 'ying shi ying di': taking into account the local diet, time of year, weather, geography, individual constitution, age, and sex.

"When the evil wind attacks people, it comes like a storm. We can map out its course of attack, beginning with the pores and skin, into the muscle layer, through the tendomuscular layer, into the vessels, and into the six fu and the five zang organs. A superior doctor arrests disease at the skin level and dispels it before it penetrates deeper. An inferior doctor treats illness after it passes the skin. If the pathogen is not stopped on the surface, it enters the muscle level and must be dispersed there. If it progresses and invades deep into the five zang organs, the prognosis for recovery is only fifty percent.

"The six exogenous pathogenic factors cause disharmonies in people by invading from the external to the internal and moving from the superficial level deep into the zang fu organs. Improper diet mainly affects the six fu organs; pathogenic dampness will cause disruption to the skin, flesh, muscles, tendons, and vessels, and will stagnate at the joints. A proficient acupuncturist must understand the principle of external and internal, disease invading from outside to inside, inside to outside, and the connections and relationships between yang and yin, qi and blood, and the channels and collaterals.

"With this knowledge it is possible to direct the pathogen from the inside to the outside, to dispel it from the outside, or move it from the outside to the inside to be purged and eliminated. When disease is on the right side, treat the left, and when it is on the left, treat the right. Compare one's normalcy with others' abnormality. When observing the condition it is possible to see what is occurring on the inside from the symptoms on the outside. The progression of the condition, its severity and prognosis, can also be ascertained.

"A doctor adept at diagnosis observes the patient's shen, complexion, facial color, and pulses. First, it must be determined whether the illness is yin or yang, then the facial colors will indicate the location of the disease, and finally the voice and breathing will confirm the nature of the suffering.

"When the abnormal pulse is compared to a normal one, it is possible to know if a pathogen is present. One must consider the variations of the normal pulses that are natural in each season. If the radial pulse at the most distal point on the wrist is floating or sinking, slippery or choppy, the cause of the imbalance will be known. Following this method, one will avoid mistakes.

"In the beginning stage of illness, while the pathogen is relatively superficial, acupuncture can be used effectively to open the surface and eliminate the pathogen. When the illness is at a raging stage, it is necessary to wait until the peak passes, then administer acupuncture for successful results. When the pathogenic factor is external and strong, one can retain the acupuncture needle longer and apply strong stimulation. This will weaken the pathogen and reinforce the zheng/antipathogenic qi, enabling it to eliminate the illness.

"When an illness is on the surface of the body, herbs that are pungent and diaphoretic can be used to disperse it. If the condition is excess and internal, purgative herbs are used to purge and eliminate it. If the zheng/antipathogenic qi is weakened, tonic herbs will fortify it. It is necessary to determine if the illness is due to yang or yin deficiency. If it is yang deficiency, warming herbs and qi tonics are appropriate, while in the case of yin deficiency, thicker, more nourishing yin and blood tonic herbs are indicated.

"The location of an illness will determine the treatment method. An illness located above the diaphragm and chest can be treated with emetics to induce vomiting, while an illness below the diaphragm and in the intestines can be purged. If it is in the middle, involving the stomach, then digestive and carminative herbs will be used. When the illness is in the skin, induce sweating to eliminate it, but if zheng/antipathogenic qi is weak, causing leakages such as diarrhea, astringent herbs will be helpful. If the qi is stuck, its movement can be restored through the use of carminative herbs; severe stagnation should be broken up with stronger herbs.

"Illness should be differentiated by the eight principles of yin or yang, internal or external, excess or deficiency, and hot or cold, so that the right method may be employed to counteract the condition and restore homeostasis. Acupuncture treatment can subdue the reckless movement of blood and qi and restore their natural and smooth flow. When a pathogen attacks the qi and blood, this is an excess condition. In this case acupuncture points can be used to induce bleeding and eliminate the pathogen. If there is a qi deficiency in a particular location or channel, the qi can be conducted or guided from other channels to supplement the weakness."

CHAPTER 6

—

THE INTERPLAY OF
YIN AND YANG

—

HUANG DI said, "I understand that heaven and the sun are considered yang, and earth and the moon are considered yin. Because of the natural movement of heaven and earth and the sun and moon, we experience a change of long months and short months and go through three hundred and sixty-five days, which form one year in the Chinese calendar. The energy flow within the human body through the channels corresponds to this. Can you elaborate further?"

Qi Bo answered, "The reaches of heaven and earth and yin and yang are vast, and ultimately everything in the universe can be classified into the polarity of yin and yang.

"Yin and yang are not absolute, but their principle never changes. The law that governs does not falter, although everything around it changes according to the point of reference. For example, before the birth of all things and creatures above ground, the living potential resided in the place of yin. This is called yin within yin. Once it was born and appeared above ground, this phenomenon was called yang within yin. It was after birth or post-heaven that the yang qi enabled everything to grow.

"Yin provides form. Yang enables growth. Warmth of the spring gives rise to birth, the fire of the summer fuels rapid growth and development, the coolness of autumn matures all and provides harvest, and the coldness of winter forces inactivity and storing. This is the rhythmic change of nature. If the four seasons become disrupted, the weather becomes unpredictable and the energies of the universe will lose their normalcy. This principle also applies to the body."

Huang Di then said, "I wish to hear you expound on the separation and the union of the three yang."

Qi Bo replied, "The sage stands facing south. In front of him is guang ming or broad expanse, in back of him is tai chong or great fall. Traveling in this lower region of tai chong is a channel called shaoyin or minor yin. Above this is the taiyang or major yang/bladder channel. The lower part of the taiyang/bladder channel begins at the outside of the small toe at the point zhiyin (B67). The upper part connects with jingming (B1) in the face near the eyes.

"The taiyang/bladder channel is coupled with the shaoyin/kidney channel. The taiyang/bladder is lateral and exposed to the sun and is considered external. The shaoyin is medial and is in the shade and is considered internal. We call this yang within yin.

"Now let us take a look at the upper part of the body. The upper is yang and is called guang ming. The lower is yin and is called taiyin or major yin. Anterior to the taiyin area is the yangming or moderate yang. The most distal point of the yangming/stomach channel ends on the tip of the second toe at the lidui (ST45) point. Because the yangming is the exterior that is exposed to the sun, relative to the taiyin, it is also called yang within yin.

"The interior of the body is yin. Just exterior to that gives rise to the minor yang, as it is gradually exposed to the sun. This is called shaoyang, which is the pivot between the interior and the exterior. The shaoyang/gallbladder channel begins at the zhuqiaoyin point (G44). Jueyin is the extreme of yin and the end of yin, and it gives birth to the beginning of yang. We call this shaoyang within yin. Now we should differentiate and summarize the three yang channels.

"Taiyang is on the surface, and its nature is open and expansive; it is the outside. The yangming is internal and its action is storing; thus it is the house. The shaoyang, which is between the internal and external, acts as a bridge and is considered the hinge between interior and exterior. The three yang, however, do not act separately, but rather in unison. So, collectively we call them one yang."

Huang Di asked, "What about the separation and the union of the three yin?" Qi Bo replied, "The outside is yang and the inside yin; that has been established. What is inside consists of the three yin. The taiyin/spleen is medial and is in the shade. This channel begins on the side of the big toe at the point yinbai (SP1). It is called yin within yin. Behind the taiyin there is the shaoyin/kidney channel, which begins at the bottom of the foot at yongchuan (K1) point. It is considered the shaoyin within yin.

"Anterior to shaoyin we have jueyin or extreme yin. The jueyin/liver channel begins on the other side of the big toe at the point dadun (LIV1). Surrounded and preceded by two yin channels, the jueyin is the most yin of the yin channels. Thus it is called jueyin of the yin, the extreme yin.

"In summary, we can say that the taiyin is the most superficial of the three yin channels, and its nature is expansive. The jueyin is the deepest inside of the yin. Its nature is that of storing and thus it is considered the house. The shaoyin is in between, and acts to connect and is considered the hinge or door. The three yin must also work in unison. Collectively, too, these are considered one yin.

"So you have one yin and one yang. The qi of the yin and of the yang move unobstructed throughout the entire body. This is because of the interplay of the yin and yang and the relationship of the exterior and interior."

CHAPTER 7

FURTHER DISCOURSE ON
YIN AND YANG

HUANG DI asked, "It is said that humans have four jing/pulses or four normally occurring pulses and twelve chong or movements. What does this mean?"

Qi Bo answered, "The four jing/pulses consist of the pulses of the four seasons, and the twelve movements correspond to the twelve channels, which in turn correspond to the twelve months of the year.

"Normally, in spring, the pulse is wiry, in summer it is flooding, in autumn it is floating, and in winter it is sinking. Additionally, in late summer, the pulse is normally moderate. These are normal signs reflecting the macrocosmic changes and are classified as yang pulses. The twelve movements reflect the qi flow in the various channels throughout the year. The hand taiyin/lung starts around February, the first month of the Chinese calendar. The hand yangming/large intestine occurs in March, the foot yangming/stomach in April, the foot taiyin/spleen in May, the hand shaoyin/heart in June, the hand taiyang/small intestine in July, the foot taiyang/bladder in August, the foot shaoyin/kidney in September, the hand jueyin/pericardium in October, the hand shaoyang/sanjiao in November, the foot shaoyang/gallbladder in December, and the foot jueyin/liver in January.

"The five normally variable yang pulses due to season and the five individual pulses of the zang organs actually combine to make up twenty-five pulses. Yang pulses reflect the health of the stomach qi.

"A yin pulse that shows no stomach qi is called the pulse of zhen zang. Zhen zang, or decaying pulse, indicates that the stomach qi is drained and exhausted and the prognosis is usually death. Why? Because a yin pulse reflects absence of yang and thus absence of life activity. If you can distinguish the presence or absence of the stomach pulse, you can know where the disease is located and give the prognosis for life or death, and even know when death might occur.

"The pulses of the three yang channels can be found next to the Adam's apple on the carotid artery, known as ren ying (ST9). The three yin pulses are detected at the radial artery on the wrist, which is called guan kou. Under healthy circumstances, the pulses of ren ying and guan kou should be identical and in harmony.

"We can also categorize each individual pulse. When the pulse arrives it is yang, and when it recedes it is yin. When the pulse is active it is yang, and when it is quiet it is yin. When the pulse is rapid it is yang. Rapid is defined as more than five beats per breath of the doctor. When the pulse is slow it is yin. Yin is defined as fewer than four beats per doctor's breath. Systolic is yang, and diastolic is yin. When the wave of the pulse goes up it is yang, and when it goes down it is yin.

"When Yang pulses are absent in a patient, the yin or the decaying pulse of the liver is like a thin thread on the verge of breaking, or like a tightly wound wire about to snap. The patient will die within eighteen days. If the decaying pulse of the heart is like a thin fragile thread, the patient will surely die in nine days. If this pulse is found in the lung pulse, the patient will not survive longer than twelve days. If it is found in the kidney pulse, the patient will die in seven days. If it is found in the spleen pulse, the patient will die in four days. Generally, disorders of the stomach and intestines affect the spleen and heart. People suffering from these imbalances have difficulty expressing their ills. In women, irregular menstruation or amenorrhea can occur. If illness lingers, emaciation will result. This is called feng xiao, dehydration and exhaustion caused by wind arising from heat. When rapid, shallow breathing occurs, with difficulty catching one's breath, or xi fen, it is considered incurable.

"Disease of the taiyang channel consists of symptoms such as fever and chills, skin lesions, boils, carbuncles, and swelling in the lower extremities. This disease may also manifest in weakness in the knees, cold and spasms with difficult movement, and soreness and pain in back of the thighs and calves.

"As the disease progresses and becomes chronic, it manifests as dryness of the skin, or it can cause swelling of the testicles or ovarian pain.

"As it transfers to the shaoyang channel, it manifests as susceptibility to cough, diarrhea, and low energy. If chronic, it can become pain in the chest due to heart deficiency or food retention with no appetite.

"Yangming and jueyin disease will most often manifest as startling, anxiety, fright, and back pain with burping, hiccuping or yawning. This can lead to Feng Jue, syncope due to wind.

"Shaoyin and shaoyang illnesses cause distension in the abdominal and epigastric areas. Then we have fullness, with possible nausea and vomiting, and also burping and hiccuping.

"When taiyang and taiyin illness occur together, we may see hemiplegia, wei condition or flaccidity, and weakness.

"But let us return to the pulses. When the pulse comes with force it is yang, and when it relaxes it is yin. When the pulse comes with much strength but then goes completely weak, this is called a flooding pulse. When the pulse arrives light and floating and slightly weak, we call it a floating pulse.

"A pulse that is full and tense, as if touching a string on the pi pa, or Chinese guitar, is called wiry. When it is full but deep, that is, upon light pressure at the superficial level you don't feel much but with strong pressure you feel it full, this is called a sinking pulse.

"A pulse that is neither too strong nor too weak, that comes and goes in a rhythmic fashion, flowing like a stream, is called a slippery or moderate pulse.

"Yin and yang are unbalanced when the yin qi is excessive and stagnant on the inside and the yang qi moves recklessly outward, with profuse sweating, cold extremities, dyspnea, and wheezing; this is dangerous because it involves the collapse of yin and yang. The transformation of yin depends on the normal balance of yin and yang. A gentle warming method is appropriate; if a harsh heating method is applied to counter the imbalance, the yang qi will be forced to escape, and the yin qi will follow it to oblivion. If the yin qi is abundant and excess, then cold and dampness will dominate and this will also stagnate blood and qi, causing death.

"There is a condition of dying yin in which the patient will not live beyond three days. An example of this can be illustrated with heart disease transferring to the lungs; in the control cycle of the five elements, this is fire dominating metal, resulting in dysfunction and subsequent death. In a condition of yang revival, the patient will recover within four days. Yang revival can be illustrated by liver disease transferring to the heart; wood creates fire, following the creative cycle of the five elemental phases, resulting in recovery.

"There are two other conditions: zhong yin, or heavy yin, in which lung disease transfers to the kidney; and pi yin, or uncontrollable yin, in which kidney disease transfers to the spleen. Both are incurable. In zhong yin, metal creates water via the creation cycle, but is lacking yang, resulting in a negative outcome; hence, zhong yin. In pi yin, water humiliates earth, a reversal of the control cycle. The yin element is dominant and out of control; thus, the result is pi yin.

"When pathogens cause obstruction within the yang channels, edema occurs. When pathogens affect the yin channels, blood in the stools results. When both yin and yang channels are obstructed, but the yin channels are more severely affected, the lower abdomen will swell; this is called shi shui. Furthermore, when the stomach and large intestine channels are more seriously obstructed, a condition of xiao ke, or diabetic exhaustion syndrome, will occur. When the bladder and small intestine channels are more affected, obstructions of bowel and urine will occur. When the spleen and lung channels are affected, abdominal edema and distension occur. When the liver and gallbladder channels are affected, throat blockage, or hou bi, results.

"When examining the pulses, if one finds the yin pulses are distinctly different from the yang pulses, this indicates pregnancy. If both yin and yang pulses are deficient and the patient has dysentery, this indicates a grave prognosis. If the yang pulses are twice as strong as the yin pulses, the patient will sweat spontaneously. If the yin pulses are deficient and the yang pulses are excessively full, the indication is excess fire causing extravasation; in women, metrorrhagia will result.

"In determining the prognosis of an illness, if the spleen and lung pulses are abnormally full, the patient will not survive beyond midnight of the twentieth day; if the heart and kidney pulses are abnormally full, the patient will not live past the evening of the thirteenth day; if the pericardium and liver pulses are abnormally full, the patient will not live longer than ten days; if the bladder and small intestine pulses are abnormally full, the patient will die within three days; if the stomach and large intestine pulses are abnormally full, particularly in febrile disease, the patient will not live beyond ten days. Finally, when all pulses are abnormally full, with epigastric and abdominal swelling or distension and obstruction of bowels and urine, the indication is that both yin and yang qi have reached the zenith of exhaustion. Consequently, the patient will not live beyond five days."

CHAPTER 8

THE SACRED TEACHINGS

HUANG DI asked Qi Bo, "Can you please tell me the functions and the relationships of the twelve zang fu viscera and their meridians?"

Qi Bo replied, "Your question is very precise and I will try to answer you as precisely as you asked. The heart is the sovereign of all organs and represents the consciousness of one's being. It is responsible for intelligence, wisdom, and spiritual transformation. The lung is the advisor. It helps the heart in regulating the body's qi. The liver is like the general, courageous and smart. The gallbladder is like a judge for its power of discernment. The pericardium is like the court jester who makes the king laugh, bringing forth joy. The stomach and spleen are like warehouses where one stores all the food and essences. They digest, absorb, and extract the food and nutrients. The large intestine is responsible for transportation of all turbidity. All waste products go through this organ. The small intestine receives the food that has been digested by the spleen and stomach and further extracts, absorbs, and distributes it throughout the body, all the while separating the pure from the turbid. The kidneys store the vitality and mobilize the four extremeties. They also aid the memory, willpower, and coordination. The sanjiao, or the three visceral cavities, promotes the transformation and transportation of water and fluids throughout the body. The bladder is where the water converges and where, after being catalyzed by the qi, it is eliminated. So these twelve zang and fu organs must work together harmoniously, just like a kingdom.

"However, the decision-making is the king's job. If the spirit is clear, all the functions of the other organs will be normal. It is in this way that one's life is preserved and perpetuated, just as a country becomes prosperous when all its people are fulfilling their duties. If the spirit is disturbed and unclear, the other organs will not function properly. This creates damage. The pathways and roads along which the qi flows will become blocked and health will suffer. The citizens of the kingdom will also suffer. These are the relationships of a kingdom."

Qi Bo continued, "The principles of healing and medicine in general are difficult to grasp because many changes occur in illness, and the healing process must adapt to that. It becomes difficult to know the root. The origin of illness can be so small and vague, in fact, so elusive, but the illness can still become substantial over time."

As Qi Bo spoke of the subtlety and difficulty of medicine and healing, Huang Di exclaimed, "Aha! I finally understand the intricacies and the essence of healing. I cannot receive this treasure carelessly. I must pick the best day and time to receive and store this knowledge. I must put this in my secret chamber and preserve it and pass it down to future generations."

CHAPTER 9

—

THE ENERGETIC CYCLES
OF THE UNIVERSE AND THEIR
EFFECTS ON HUMAN BEINGS

—

Huang Di asked, "I have heard that in the heavenly realm, cycles of energy are composed of six sixty-day cycles, which create one year. On earth this is also measured by the nine continents and nine orifices, referred to as the 'rule of nine.' The combination of the six cycles and the rule of nine produces the three hundred and sixty-five days that make one year. There are three hundred and sixty-five energy points in the human body that are in concert with the philosophy with the human being as a microcosm of the macrocosmic universe. This kind of correspondence extrapolation has been in use for a long time; however, I am ignorant of its reasons."

Qi Bo replied, "You have asked a very intelligent question. I will tell you everything about this. The six cycles and the rule of nine are used to measure the energy flow in the year and the degree of travel of the sun and moon in relation to the earth. The changes in heaven determine the birth and death of all things on earth.

"Heaven above is yang and earth below is yin. The sun travels during the day in the heavens and is yang. The moon travels in the evening and is yin. There is a regular rhythm of movement to the sun and moon, and specific pathways that have been mapped out from ancient times. The earth makes a complete revolution around the sun in exactly one year, and it rotates exactly once before the sun in one day and one night. The moon moves a little more than thirteen degrees around the earth on a daily basis. Since ancient times, each month is determined by the waxing and waning of the moon. This is why we have 'large months' and 'small months' in the lunar calendar. To start one must accurately determine at the beginning of the year the commencement of the first cycle. This is done by planting a stick straight into the ground and measuring the shadows of the stick throughout the day and the year in relation to the sun. This will enable us to map out twenty-four solar terms accurately throughout the season."

Huang Di said further, "Now I understand the measurements of heaven. I would like to further understand the interactions between the measurement of heaven and the cycles of change that govern the earth which apply to human beings."

Qi Bo answered, "Heaven is measured by the rules of six, and earth and human beings are governed by the rule of nine. The sages of ancient time carefully observed the heavens and noted their surroundings, and proposed a complex system, consisting of several subsystems to account for all possible variables, in the forecast of macrocosmic influence upon the world; especially the weather and the effects on people.

"The basic building blocks of this complex system utilize representative symbols of the ten heavenly stems and the twelve earthly branches, each symbol representing an aspect of the natural process of the universe. The combination of the stems and the branches produces a cycle of sixty which is applied to keeping track of time. Each year in the Chinese calendar is divided into twenty-four fortnightly segments called jie qi, or solar terms. Four terms equal sixty days and is called a bu or step. Six steps makes up a year. In a sixty-year cycle, there are all together one thousand and four hundred and forty solar terms. Since ancient times, one who understands this system would have mastery of all the processes in the universe, because everything that is living has an intimate association with this change in heavenly energy circulation. This is due to the interaction with heaven's yang and earth's yin and the qi to carry out the process of birth, growth, maturation, and death.

The phases of the five elements and atmospheric influences in nature all have their peak flows during different times of the year. At year's end, this begins over again. This continues in a cycle ad infinitum. Therefore, if a person does not grasp and understand the year's energy flow, the peaks and valleys of the qi, the excesses and deficiencies of the body, and the pathogens, that person does not qualify to become a doctor."

Huang Di said, "Now I understand the energetic cycles throughout the seasons and within the five elements or phases. But I am still slightly baffled by the excesses and deficiencies during the process of energy transformation."

Qi Bo replied, "All the changes and transformations through the five parts of the year—spring, summer, late summer, autumn, and winter—have their excesses and deficiencies. This is a normal process."

Huang Di asked, "How do you achieve balance or even flow between each season?"

Qi Bo replied, "It means neither extreme in weather patterns and hence the effect on people."

Huang Di said, "Can you explain what constitutes an even cyclic flow?"

Qi Bo answered, "This is recorded in the ancient books."

Huang Di asked, "What is meant by control or dominance of excessive energy?"

Qi Bo replied, "This means when a seasonal attribute abnormally dominates during another season. For instance, spring controls late summer. Late summer controls winter. Winter controls summer. Summer controls autumn. And autumn controls spring. This is the control cycle in the transformation process of the five elemental phases. These abnormal occurrences in nature negatively affect the human body and its corresponding five zang organs. The wood element of spring corresponds to the liver, the summer element of fire corresponds to the heart; the late summer element of earth corresponds to the spleen, the autumn element of metal corresponds to the lungs, and the winter element of water corresponds to the kidneys."

Huang Di asked, "How do we predict when an element or season will control another, and what can we gain from this knowledge?"

Qi Bo answered, "In order to utilize the knowledge of the five elemental phases, one must first calculate the time of the arrival of the seasons and observe the normal and abnormal patterns. Generally, we would calculate from the first day of spring in the Chinese calendar. If the first day of spring has not arrived, but the weather or the atmospheric influence are warming, we consider this to be an excess of fire. This fire excess would then humiliate the water element and damage the normalcy of the season. It would further overcontrol the normal qi of metal. This is called qi ying, or reckless qi. In this case, disease of the kidneys and lungs would manifest. On the other hand, if the first day of the season has arrived, but the warming weather trend and the atmospheric influence have not arrived, this is considered to be fire deficiency. This fire deficiency is unable to control the original weather patterns and causes the originally controlled element to be unrestrained. Further, the water element would gain strength and cause the fire to be weakened. If the fire is weakened the earth cannot produce, and a disease pattern mirroring this imbalance will manifest. As a result of this deficiency the body or seasonal qi is invaded. This is called qi po, meaning suppression or deficient qi. Through careful observation of the time of the season and the arrival of the appropriate weather and cyclic patterns, we can understand and apply the knowledge of the transformation of the five elements. Thus, a doctor who does not understand or has misinterpreted the peaks and valleys of the cycles of nature will not understand the mechanism by which people get sick. That doctor will be ineffective in both the treatment and the prognosis of patients."

Huang Di asked, "In this five-elemental circuit throughout the seasons, do normal changes and transformations ever not follow their proper order?"

Qi Bo answered, "In nature, the cyclic flow through the five seasons cannot afford to become disordered, because without order, injury and even death can occur."

Huang Di asked, "How then does it become abnormal and how does this manifest?"

Qi Bo replied, "This abnormality of the five elemental phases circuit can cause illness in people. For example, if in spring we have the weather patterns of late summer, or dampness, this corresponds to wood controlling earth. This illness is considered to be mild, because it is one of overcontrol. If in spring we find the dry, cool weather of fall, this becomes metal attacking wood. In this case the illness would be severe, because it results in a deficiency. If, at the same time, other pathogens come into play, there may be the possibility of death. When abnormal weather patterns occur in nature and are not invasive, the problem is light. When they are invasive or attacking, the illness can become quite severe."

Huang Di said, "I have heard that all things in nature derive their form from the qi of heaven and earth. Because the qi of heaven and earth transforms and changes and is so variable, the forms of nature and living things are also variable. Can you further expound on this and the changes of yin and yang, heaven and earth, and the energetic phases of the environment and how these determine what will prosper and what will diminish?"

Qi Bo said, "You have asked a very detailed question. Because of its vastness, the universe is difficult to measure. Your question is of tremendous depth. I do not think I can adequately detail my answer. But I can give you a generalization.

"In the plant kingdom there are the five colors. Within the five colors there are variations in tone. The plants have five flavors. Though distinct, there are also variations of the flavors. The five colors and five flavors correspond to and affect the five zang organs of the body. Heaven provides yang as qi and provides for people the five colors, while earth, being yin and substantial, provides people with five flavors. The five qi, or colors, can also be said to be absorbed through the nose as the five fragrances. These are stored in the heart and lungs. The heart is responsible for manifesting the facial colors and the lungs are responsible for producing sound. The five flavors enter through the mouth and are stored in the stomach and intestines. After the digestion and the absorption of nourishment, this qi is used to enhance the function of the five zang organs. The qi of the five zang organs combines with the qi of the five flavors to produce the jin and ye/body fluids, which lubricate and further fortify the body, marrow, and jing/essence. These naturally support a vigorous shen/spirit."

Huang Di asked, "How do the functional aspects of the zang organs manifest outwardly?"

Qi Bo answered, "Heart is the root of life and the seat of shen or intelligence. It manifests its prosperity on the face, because of its function of keeping the blood vessels full. It is located above the diaphragm and is considered to be yang. Its element is fire. Therefore, it is called the taiyang of the yang. In the universal pattern flow it corresponds to the summer. The lungs, being the roots of the body's qi, dominate qi. They store po/ courage. They manifest their abundance in the body hair, and their function is to maintain the fullness and suppleness of the skin. The lungs are the highest organs in the body, and their element is metal. They are considered the taiyin within the yang, and they correspond to autumn energy. The kidneys are the storage place of the true yang and the root of all storage in the body. They store the jing/essence qi of the five zang and six fu organs. They manifest their abundance and health in the head hair. Its effect is to fill the bones and marrow. Being a water element in the lower trunk, the kidneys are considered yin. They are called the shaoyin of the yin and correspond to the winter energy. The liver is the reservoir of stamina, storing the hun/intuition. It manifests in the nails, and functions in strengthening the tendons. It stores blood. The liver is in the yin location of the abdomen, but belongs to the yang element of wood. It is thus called the shaoyang of yin. It corresponds with the spring.

The stomach, small intestine, large intestine, bladder, and sanjiao are also all receptors and storehouses of water and food. They are the producers of ying or nutritive qi. They absorb the essence from water and food, transport them properly, and eliminate waste and turbidity. They are able to transform the five flavors of food, and they manifest their health in the lips and mouth. They are responsible for keeping full the flesh and muscles. They are all located in the abdomen and are responsible for taking in and storing the turbid yin of the five flavors and substances. They collectively assist the functions of the spleen organ. They are considered to be extreme yin and correspond to late summer and the earth element. Therefore, we consider the spleen to be extreme yin within yin. The zang and fu organs that I have described are all dependent on the functions of the gallbladder and its decision-making. The gallbladder corresponds to spring, initiation, and decisiveness. When the gallbladder qi is properly ascended and dispersed, the other eleven organs can easily function in health and prosperity.

"When the carotid pulse is twice as large as normal, the illness is in the beginning stage of heat and is located in shaoyang. When it is three times as large, the illness is in the middle stage of heat and resides in taiyang. When it is four times as large, the illness is in a severe stage of heat and is in yangming. When it is five times as large, the yang has escaped to the outside.

"When the radial pulse is twice as large as normal, the illness is in the beginning stage of cold and is in jueyin. When it is three times as large, the illness is in mid-stage of cold and resides in shaoyin. When it is four times as large, the illness is in the severe stage of cold and is in taiyin. When it is five times as large, the yin has collapsed. If both the carotid and radial pulses are five times larger than normal, this condition is called guan ke or obstructed. This means that yin and yang have become extreme and stagnant, and collapse is imminent. The prenatal and postnatal jing/essence qi have become exhausted, and the eventual consequence is death."

CHAPTER 10

—

DYSFUNCTION OF THE FIVE ZANG VISCERA

—

Qi Bo began by saying, "The vessels correspond with the heart, which manifests its essence in the facial complexion. However, the heart is controlled by the kidneys. The skin corresponds with the lungs, which manifest their essence in the body hair. However, the lungs are controlled by the heart. The tendons correspond with the liver, which manifests its essence in the nails and is controlled by the lungs. The flesh and muscles correspond with the spleen, which manifests its essence on the lips and is controlled by the liver. The bones and marrow correspond with the kidneys, which manifest in the head hair and are controlled by the spleen.

"Overindulgence in salty foods will coagulate the blood circulation and will change the color of the blood. Overindulgence in bitter food will cause the skin to become shriveled and dry and the body hair to fall out. Overindulgence in pungent food can cause spasms, tremors, and poor nails. Overly excessive consumption of sour foods can make the skin rough, thick, and wrinkled, and cause the lips to become shriveled. Overindulgence in sweets will cause pain in the bones and hair loss. All these symptoms and conditions are a result of overindulgence of the five flavors.

"It is said that the heart is benefited by the bitter taste, the lung by the pungent taste, the spleen by the sweet taste, the liver by the sour taste, and the kidneys by the salty taste. However, this never implies that one may overindulge.

"The qi of the five zang organs manifests in the face. If we see green as in the color of a dying plant, or if we see yellow similar to *Fructus ponceri*, or if we see black as in ashes, as in stuck, bruising, coagulated blood, or white as in bones, these are the colors of death. If we see green like jade, red like the crown of a rooster, yellow like the underside of a crab, white like the lard of a pig, or black like the feathers of a black chicken, these are the colors of life.

"So the color that benefits the heart is similar to a white silk cloth wrapped around cinnabar. The color that produces liver qi is like white silk wrapping a green color. The spleen color would be a white handkerchief wrapping *Fructus trichosanthis,* and for the kidney it is the handkerchief wrapping the color purple. These are all normal colors or complexions of the face.

"The five colors and the five tastes correspond to the five zang organs. So we can say that the white color and pungent taste correspond to the lungs, red and bitter correspond to the heart, green and sour to the liver, yellow and sweet to the spleen, and black and salty to the kidneys. We can additionally say that white corresponds to the skin, red to the vessels, green to the tendons, yellow to the flesh, and black to the bones.

"The jing, the essence of the five zang and six fu, the twelve channels and collaterals, all converge in the eyes, while all marrow converges in the brain. All the tendons connect the bones and joints. All the blood and body fluids are controlled by the heart, all the qi by the lungs. The four extremities and the twelve joints are the highways of the channels, marrow, tendons, blood, and qi.

"The liver stores blood. During the day the liver provides the blood for movement and activities, so that the blood can circulate throughout the channels and collaterals. At night, when one sleeps, the blood returns to the liver. When the liver is nourished by the blood, one can see. When the feet are perfused with blood, one can walk. When the hands are nourished by blood, they can grasp. When the fingers are provided with blood, one can carry.

"All disorders can be attributed to the blood and qi not arriving at certain streams and valleys and caves, an analogy of acupoints. Then, the pathogenic wind has an opportunity to invade and cause bi/obstruction syndrome and spasms.

"In the body we have twelve spaces between the muscles where the energy flows, and many small convergences of energy at small spaces between muscles, excluding the twelve shu/stream points. These are all locations where the wei/defensive qi accumulates to protect the body. At the same time, these places are also doors and windows through which the evil wind or pathologic factors can enter. That is why, if these points are invaded by the evil wind, acupuncture can be used to dispel it from these doors and windows. To become proficient in diagnosis, one must utilize the pulses of the five zang organs as a base. To truly grasp and understand the pulses of the five zang organs, one must understand etiology.

"If one suffers from a headache in the upper part of the head, it is because there is an excess in the upper and a deficiency in the lower. The disease is in the foot shaoyin/kidney and foot taiyang/bladder. If the illness worsens, it can transfer to the liver, causing dizziness, vertigo, blurry vision, and deafness. This would be a reversal, with deficiency in the upper part and excess in the lower. Now the channels affected are foot shaoyang/gallbladder and foot jueyin/liver.

"If the illness further worsens, it transfers to the spleen, resulting in distension in the abdomen, chest fullness, and pain in the ribs. This is because the qi is stuck in the lower part and cannot rise to the upper part of the body. In this case, the stagnation is residing in the foot taiyin/spleen and foot yangmeng/stomach.

"When we have cough, asthma, difficulty breathing, and chest fullness and distension, this is because the illness manifests in the hand yangmeng/large intestines and hand taiyin/lung channels. When we have irritability and headache and an obstructed feeling in the diaphragm, this is because the illness manifests in the hand taiyang and shaoyin channels.

"The characteristics of the pulses, such as small, large, slippery, choppy, floating, and sinking, can be detected and differentiated with the three fingers. It is through the detection of the subtle changes that we can correctly see the condition of the five zang organs.

"The five zang organs correspond to the five sounds, and we can diagnose through the five sounds. We can also observe the five colors, and see the essences of the organs through the five colors. If we can combine the colors, the sounds, and the pulses together to differentiate, the picture becomes complete.

"So, if we see redness and simultaneously a rapid and wiry pulse, we know this is because the qi is stuck at zhongwan (REN12), the epigastrium. This causes problems with digestion and a condition called xing bi, or bi/obstruction of the heart.

"Heart bi syndrome is not limited to joint problems. It can also be caused by invasion of an exterior pathogen. This might be because the heart qi is weakened from excessive thinking and worry and the body has become vulnerable, allowing the pathogen to invade the epigastrium, causing the qi to become stuck.

"If we see a white color on the face, and at the same time the pulse is rapid, floating, and empty, deficient in the upper and excessive in the lower, and the patient has anxiety with spasms, this is because the qi is stuck in the chest. This is asthma and lung deficiency. The lung deficiency is called lung bi/obstruction of the lungs, and the cause is drinking wine and indulging in sexual activities afterward.

"If we see green and the pulse is long and wiry, this is because the qi is stuck under the epigastrium, underneath the ribs and hypochondriac area. This is called liver bi and is due to invasion of cold and dampness; it is similar to the pathology of hernias. Thus, one will have back pain, headache, and cold feet.

"If we see a yellow color and the pulse is large and deficient, this is because the qi is stuck in the abdominal area because of spleen deficiency, with kidney qi rebelling upward. This causes stagnant qi, and later, hiatal hernia.

"If we see black and the pulse is hard and large, this is because the qi is stuck in the lower abdomen just above the genitals. This is kidney bi and can result from taking a shower just before going to sleep.

"Through the five colors, we can diagnose properly. If we observe a yellow color in the face and green eyes, or a yellow face with red eyes, or a yellow face with white eyes, or a yellow face with black eyes, these are all considered symptoms of nonfatal disharmonies. But if the face turns green and the eyes turn red, or if the face is red and the eyes white, or the face is green and the eyes black, or the face is black and the eyes are white, or the face red and the eyes green, these are all signs of death.

"This is because when the face is yellow the spleen qi still nourishes, but when the face turns another color nourishing has stopped, and death will occur."

CHAPTER 11

—

FURTHER DISCOURSE ON THE FIVE ZANG VISCERA

—

Huang Di asked, "I have heard from scholars the different explanations and classification of the zang and fu organs. Some feel that the brain and marrow, the large intestine and the small intestine are zang. Others feel that these are fu. People all disagree. I would like to hear from you a clarification on the correct classification."

Qi Bo replied, "The brain, marrow, bones, blood vessels, gallbladder, and uterus are all born of the earthly qi. Similar to the earthly function, they store. They store essence. So they are considered extraordinary fu organs. They are hollow containers that store substantial substances. On the other hand, the stomach, large and small intestines, sanjiao, and bladder are formed by the heavenly qi. Their function, like that of the heavenly circulation of continuous flow, is to transport rather than store. They receive the turbid qi from the five zang. Thus, they are named the palaces of transportation. They receive the food, water, and turbid qi, which cannot remain for long, and then transport such 'acquired jing' to the five zang organs, and pass on the waste products. Even the hunmen, or rectum, works by eliminating, so that the waste does not become stored in the body. Such storage would be in opposition to the principles of the six fu, and disease would then manifest. Thus, the five zang organs store the essence of jing/essence qi. They do not transport. On the other hand, the six fu organs receive the food and digest, absorb, and transport it, passing it on. They are often full, but still do not store. Food enters the mouth and proceeds to the stomach. The stomach is now full, but the intestines are empty. The foodstuff passes downward, filling the intestines. Now the stomach is empty. That is why it is said that the six fu are full but never filled, and the five zang organs are filled but never full."

Huang Di further inquired, "From palpating the pulse at the radial position, how can one know the subtleties and conditions of the five zang organs?"

Qi Bo answered, "The stomach is the sea of nutrients, the fountain of the six fu organs. All foodstuff enters the mouth and passes to the stomach. From here, the action of the spleen transforms the foodstuff into pure essence, which nourishes the five zang organs. The spleen, the foot taiyin, is responsible for the distribution of the jin and ye or body fluids. Its corresponding hand taiyin channel, the lung, is responsible for dispersing the qi. The taiyuan (LU9) point, located on the hand taiyin channel, is the influential point for the pulses. It governs the pulses. Therefore, the five zang organs and six fu organs derive their qi and nutrition from the stomach. Their corresponding strengths are reflected in the pulses. At the same time, the five smells enter the nose and are stored in the heart and lung. These are really the five qi of environmental energy that we breathe in. If illness occurs in the heart or lung, it will manifest in the nose.

"In healing, one must inquire closely as to the state of the patient's elimination, differentiate the pulse patterns, and observe accurately the patient's emotional, psychological, and spiritual states and other physical manifestations. If a patient is superstitious and does not believe in medicine, or if a patient refuses to be treated by acupuncture, or if a patient refuses any treatment, then no matter what the practitioner does, the patient will not get well. This is evidence that healing actually comes from within."

CHAPTER 12

METHODS OF TREATMENT

—

HUANG DI asked, "When doctors treat conditions, even though they may be illnesses of the same nature, they use different methods and techniques. But they all succeed. Why is this?"

Qi Bo replied, "This is because of differences or variables in geography, weather, lifestyle, and diet. For example, the east is the direction of the birth of heaven and earth. The weather there is mild, and it is close to the water. Many varieties of fish and salts can be found, so the local people eat many kinds of fish and like the salty flavor. But because they eat so much fish, which is considered a hot food, heat accumulates and stagnates in the body. They also eat too much salt, which dries, exhausts, and drains the blood. This is why people of the east often have dark skin. The commonly suffered illnesses are boils and carbuncles. The treatment of this disease often utilizes needles made of stone, which are thicker, and bleeding, which releases the heat. Thus, the method of stone needles comes from the east.

"In the west, many mountains and plateaus and thousands of miles of desert produce a wide variety of metals or ores. This natural environment is similar to the season of autumn. It has an astringent, or conserving, nature. The natives here live naturally and simply by the mountains. They are not concerned about their clothing; they wear wool and sleep on straw mats. They eat food that is often heavy, such as meats and fatty milk and cheese products. Thus they are usually obese people. Externally they are not easily invaded, because they are strong. That is why their illnesses tend to be internal. So the treatment for them is herbal. It can be said, therefore, that herbal treatment comes from the west.

"In the north we have high mountains. The majestic energy of solemn solitude is similar to the season of winter, where the atmosphere is one of calm and reserve. The weather is cold and snowy. Native people here are often nomadic and live amidst nature, exposed to the weather. Their diet also consists of meat and milk products. In this environment, their internal organs are often invaded by cold, and their conditions are excess and distended. The proper method of treating these conditions is moxibustion. It is therefore said that the method of moxibustion comes from the north.

"In the southern regions the weather is hot, and the yang qi is at its utmost. The geography consists of low mountains and valleys. Fog and mist often converge here. The local people like to eat sour and overly ripe foods, such as fruit. Their skin often shows redness. Conditions common in these areas are spasms, numbness, paralysis, bi/arthralgia syndrome, and wei/flaccidity syndrome. The correct treatment employs very fine needles. Thus, the art of the nine types of needles comes from the south. These are metal needles.

"In the center are flatlands, which are often damp. Many varieties of foods abound, and living is peaceful. Conditions that manifest most are colds, influenza, cold and heat conditions, wei/flaccidity syndromes, and atrophy. One should utilize Dao-in exercise, manipulation, adjustment, tuina, and massage. It is said therefore that Dao-in exercise and manipulation come from the center of China.

"A superior doctor is able to gather all techniques and use them either together or separately, to flexibly adapt to a changing environment, lifestyle, and geography, and to consider many variables in the treatment of a condition. Thus, it is understood that even though treatment methods are different, all can succeed in healing a condition. This is dependent on the ability of the doctor to consider all variables and select the proper principle of treatment."

CHAPTER 13

—

TREATMENT OF THE MIND
AND THE BODY

—

HUANG DI asked, "I have heard that in ancient times, when the sages treated, all they had to do was employ methods to guide and change the emotional and spiritual state of a person and redirect the energy flow. The sages utilized a method called zhu yuo, prayer, ceremony, and shamanism, which healed all conditions. Today, however, when doctors treat a patient, they use herbs to treat the internal aspect and acupuncture to treat the exterior. Yet some conditions do not respond. Why is this?"

Qi Bo answered, "In ancient times, people lived simply. They hunted, fished, and were with nature all day. When the weather cooled, they became active to fend off the cold. When the weather heated up in summer, they retreated to cool places. Internally, their emotions were calm and peaceful, and they were without excessive desires. Externally, they did not have the stress of today. They lived without greed and desire, close to nature. They maintained jing shen nei suo, or inner peace and concentration of the mind and spirit. This prevented the pathogens from invading. Therefore, they did not need herbs to treat their internal state, nor did they need acupuncture to treat the exterior. When they did contract disease they simply guided properly the emotions and spirit and redirected the energy flow, using the method of zhu yuo to heal the condition.

"People today are different. Internally, they are enslaved by their emotions and worries. They work too hard in heavy labor. They do not follow the rhythmic changes of the four seasons and thus become susceptible to the invasion of the thieves or winds. When their zheng/antipathogenic qi is weak, pathogens invade to destroy the five zang organs, the bones, and the marrow. Externally, they are attacked via the sensory orifices, the skin, and muscles. Thus mild conditions become severe, and severe conditions turn fatal. At this point, the method of zhu yuo would be insufficient."

Huang Di said, "Very good. However, I would like to be able to consult patients clinically in order to refine my diagnostic techniques. Then I could shed light on illness by accurately predicting prognosis as the sun and the moon illuminate the earth. I would like my mind to be illuminated. Can you tell me more about this?"

Qi Bo answered, "In diagnosis, observation of the spirit and facial color, and palpation of the pulses, are the two methods that were emphasized by the ancient emperors and revered teachers. In very ancient times there was a doctor named Jiu Dai Ji. It was he who researched the principles and techniques of observation and palpating the pulses. He was able to connect the dynamic changes of the five elements, the four seasons, the eight winds, and the six atmospheres. By doing so he was able to analyze and find the Tao from within him. If we can understand the key principles, we can readily utilize these diagnostic techniques.

"The colors and the spirit are just like the sun, which has its bright days and its cloudy days. The pulses are similar to the moon, which waxes and wanes. The signs of the pulses and observation of the colors are the keys to proper diagnosis.

"The changes in the facial complexion and the spirit have much to do with the four seasons. In the old days, the ancient virtuous emperors truly understood and utilized these principles and avoided the 'cloudy days' of their lives, thereby preserving their longevity. These emperors lived long and healthy lives and were revered as sage kings by those who came later.

"In the middle ages, prior to the Yellow Emperor's era, doctors treated differently from those of later times. When an illness occurred, they would utilize herb wines for the first ten days to eliminate the eight winds and the five bi pathogens. If after ten days the condition still persisted, they would use herbs. If they were able to grasp the etiology and pathology of a condition and work effectively to resolve the imbalance, the condition would be healed.

"But today, doctors deviate from this. They cannot even follow the changes in the four seasons. They do not know the importance and principles of the complexion and pulses. They cannot differentiate the progression and direction of a pathogen or illness. They wait until the illness has manifested itself, then they decide to use acupuncture to treat the exterior and herbs to treat the interior. They are not refined; they are sloppy. In fact, they think they can use methods of purging or sedation, not knowing that the illness has already manifested itself. It will not be healed simply by purging it out of the body, because the original cause is not removed. At the same time, many complications arise due to inaccurate treatments."

Huang Di continued his questioning. "I would be very thankful to hear some of the essentials in regard to clinical situations."

Qi Bo answered, "The key to accurate diagnosis of conditions lies in observation of the patient's color and complexion, and palpation of the pulses. These two techniques are the essential tools of diagnosis. If one does not understand and cannot utilize them, when one attempts to treat a condition, malpractice and further injury to the patient will occur. You see, if this same thing were applied to running a country, what would happen to the country? So, doctors of today should eliminate their bad habits and ignorance, open their minds, and learn the essence of pulse and color diagnosis. Only by doing so will they ever succeed in reaching the level of the ancient sages."

Huang Di said, "I have now heard you in your teachings. What you seem to be saying is that in diagnosis one should never minimize the value of the techniques of pulse and color. But are there any other specifics that one can utilize?"

Qi Bo answered, "Yes. There is one other important thing. That is the interrogation of the patient, the inquiry."

Huang Di asked, "How does one go about this?"

Qi Bo replied, "First, select a quiet environment. Close all doors and windows. Gain the trust of the patient so that the patient can completely convey everything that is pertinent to the condition. Be thorough and differentiate the truth. Observe the patient's spirit. When there is spirit, the prognosis is positive. When the spirit is gone, the condition is very grave."

CHAPTER 14

—

THE ART OF MEDICINE

—

Huang Di asked, "How are teas and wines made from the five grains?"

Qi Bo answered, "Teas and wines were all originally made from grains, mainly rice, and its stalks were used as fuel in cooking the grains. The teas were drunk or left to ferment into wine. This is how the process began. The grains, such as rice and barley, absorbed the essence from the qi of heaven and earth, and were also benefited by the harmonious manifestations of the four seasons. When they were produced in this perfect environment, they were neither too hot nor too cold. They were harvested in the autumn for the best quality. This is how wine and teas and food used to be made or prepared.

"In very ancient times, people made these herbal wines and extracts for disease prevention purposes. However, because they lived in accord with nature and followed the universal law, they were strong, knew the secrets of health preservation, and rarely got sick. So they rarely had to use them. They were made and used as a backup but were rarely necessary.

"In the middle ages, people lost the natural way. They no longer knew the correct way to live. Exterior pathogens invaded the body more easily, although people were still relatively strong. People then took herb wines and cured their diseases. However, modern patients who utilize only herb wines will not be able to get well. The reason is that nowadays people absolutely disregard the principles of healthful living. Their bodies are weaker, and illnesses come more easily and are more complex. Now many different techniques must be utilized to treat the inside and the outside. These techniques include herbs, acupuncture, moxibustion, and so forth. You now must also use poison to treat properly, because illnesses have become so compound.

Huang Di asked, "Why is it that after using all these treatment modalities, the body is still weak, the qi and blood are still deficient, and the patient does not recover?"

Qi Bo answered, "To completely heal a person, acupuncture, herbs, and these other modalities are only one aspect of the treatment. You must also come into synchrony with the patient in many other ways. For example, when patients lack the confidence to conquer illness, they allow their spirits to scatter and wither away. They let their emotions take control of their lives. They spend their days drowned in desires and worries, exhausting their jing/essence and qi and shen/spirit. Of course, then, even with all these other modalities, the disease will not be cured."

Huang Di then said, "When an illness begins, it is on a superficial level and is not complicated. The exterior pathogen will first invade from the skin level. At this stage, it is easy to cure. But illnesses today are all regarded as severe, progressing all the way to the terminal stage. Why is it that physicians who know the theories and principles of treatment, even physicians who are relatives of the patient, who hear their patients' voices and see their colors each day, why is it that these doctors do not discover illness before it occurs and treat it before it has a chance to manifest?"

Qi Bo replied, "This tells us about the level of competence of today's physicians. A good healer cannot depend on skill alone. He must also have the correct attitude, sincerity, compassion, and a sense of responsibility. The patient must also be aware of his or her body in order to recognize signs and symptoms and imbalances. That patient can then seek remedies at the earliest possible moment. When doctor and patient are in a state of harmony, the illness will not linger or become terminal."

Huang Di then said, "Some pathogenic factors do not invade at the skin level. They may come from yang deficiency of the five zang organs. When the yang is deficient, the qi cannot propel the flow of the water, and thus water is retained in the skin, causing edema. When the yang of the five zang is depleted, the yin will then take advantage and overflow in the body. This causes the qi to escape to the exterior, and the body swells even further. The extremities become very swollen. The trunk also retains water. How does one address this problem?"

Qi Bo answered, "When treating water metabolism imbalances, one must consider the degree of severity and the location of the area affected. Overall, the general treatment principle is to promote qi flow, remove stagnation, and use diuresis to get rid of excess water. First, you must move the extremities via exercise so that the yang qi can begin to flow again. Second, the patient must keep warm to prevent the yang qi from going to the superficial level to protect the body. Then acupuncture can be used to stimulate the channels and collaterals to promote the flow of yang qi again. Thus water can be regulated and metabolized, and the body will gradually return to its original state.

"At this stage, we can implement techniques of diuresis and diaphoresis. At the same time we can use herbs to fortify and strengthen the qi. Through this method, the yang qi of the five zang organs can be restored to normalcy and good circulation, returning water metabolism to normal, and eliminating pathogens. Thus yin and yang will become balanced again."

Huang Di said, "Thank you."

CHAPTER 15

—

DOCTRINES OF THE JADE TABLET

—

HUANG DI asked, "I've heard that the method of duo du qi heng, or differentiation of illness, has many applications. How would one use it?"

Qi Bo answered, "In general, duo du is used to measure the severity and depth of the illness. Qi heng is used to differentiate the nature of the illness. Let me explain from the perspective of clinical application. We start with the complexion, spirit, and pulses. When we observe the five colors and the changes in the pulses, what we are looking for is whether there is any shen/spirit or qi. The qi and blood in the human body are similar to the four seasons. They continue to flow and move forward. If they flow backward, we lose all chance of life. This is a very important principle. On one level, merely feeling the pulses and looking at the colors is superficial. But the real subject we are after is one's shen/spirit and qi.

"The five colors will manifest their significance on different parts of the face. From the relative degree of the color—deep or pale—we can surmise the characteristic of the illness. For example, if we see pale, light colors, illness is still in the beginning stage. By using food and herbal teas, the patient will be fine within ten days. If the color is deep, the illness is severe. Now strong herbs must be used, and the process may take twenty-one days. If the color is very deep, the condition is very severe. Now we have to use herb wines, which will take one hundred days to succeed. If the face is emaciated and the shen/spirit is withered, in one hundred days the patient will die. If the pulse is short and rapid and the yang qi is collapsing, one will also die. If in febrile disease, when the zheng/antipathogenic qi is extremely deficient, the patient will also die.

"Let us also discuss the movement of the color of the face. We must clearly observe such changes. If the color moves upward, this is considered rebellious. If the color moves downward, this is considered in the flow of healing. In females, if the abnormal color appears on the right side, this is considered rebellious. If it appears on the left side, it is healing. In males it is just the opposite. If the shift in colors goes from the right side to the left on a male, or the reverse on a female, this indicates an extreme imbalance of yin and yang and a grave prognosis. At this point one must utilize the techniques of duo du qi heng to measure the depth of the illness and differentiate the symptoms. Then appropriate methods must be used to correct the situation or the patient may die."

Qi Bo continued, "The pulse is an indication of the struggle between the body and the pathogen. When the pulse is irregular, this tells us that the pathogen is strong and the antipathogenic qi is weak. This can also be bi/arthralgia syndrome as in arthritic conditions, or bi syndromes where one cannot walk. This is when heat and cold are struggling in the body. If we feel the pulse is gu jue, solitary pulse, this indicates that the yang qi is exhausted. If the pulse is weak and deficient, and at the same time the patient has diarrhea, the yin and blood are injured. In general, if we see the gu pulse the prognosis is not good. If the pulse is only weak and deficient the patient can be saved.

"In diagnosis, utilizing qi heng for differentiation, beginning with the taiyin pulse at the radial artery, we can discern the reference of the four seasons and five elements. When we see that the pulse has an autumnal quality in the spring, that is, floating instead of wiry, or if we see a sinking pulse in summer instead of flooding, this tells us that the five elemental phases are out of balance. We call this rebelliousness and the prognosis is not good. If the pulse flows in its natural cycle, that is, we see a pulse of only the following season, such as autumnal pulse in summer, the condition can be cured. The relationship between the eight winds and four seasons, the flow between one season and another, will all determine the normal pulses in the body. If the four seasons become disorderly, we cannot use this to our diagnostic advantage. One who knows the meaning of this can grasp the principle of duo du qi heng."

CHAPTER 16

—

DIAGNOSTIC IMPORTANCE AND DISCUSSION OF THE COLLAPSE OF THE MERIDIANS

—

HUANG DI asked, "What are the essentials of clinical diagnosis?"

Qi Bo answered, "The most important element in clinical diagnosis is to know the relationships between heaven, earth, and humankind. For example, during February and March, the first and second months of the Chinese lunar calendar, the heavenly qi begins to rise and the earthly qi begins to germinate. In the human body, the qi is predominantly in the liver. In the third and fourth months, April and May, the heavenly qi is moderately full and the earthly qi begins to solidify. In the body, the qi is fullest in the spleen. During the fifth and sixth months, June and July, the heavenly qi becomes extremely abundant. The earthly qi now ascends. In the body, the qi rises to the head. In the seventh and eighth months, August and September, we have a turning point. The heavenly qi descends and disperses while the earthly qi consolidates. In the body, the qi is now in the lungs. In the ninth and tenth months, October and November, the heavenly qi is quiescent while the earthly qi is full, and deepens. Now freezing occurs. At this point, the qi is in the heart. In the eleventh and twelfth months, December and January, the heavenly qi is dormant and the earthly qi is completely crystallized and solid. In the body, the qi is now in the kidney.

"The qi of the body flows in accordance with the changes of heaven and earth. Therefore, when one administers acupuncture during the spring, it is appropriate to needle shu points. In fact, bloodletting is a preferred technique. If the illness is severe, one should leave the needles in longer to allow the qi to spread throughout. If it is a superficial or mild condition, one should allow the qi to circulate through all meridians of the body one time before removing the needles. This takes approximately thirty minutes. In the summer one can also practice bloodletting, but it is preferable to use superficial luo/collateral connecting points. Allow the bleeding to stop by itself, so that the pathogen will be completely eliminated. Then press on the acupuncture point and wait for the energy to circulate one time throughout the body. In this manner pain can be alleviated. In the autumn, one should concentrate on skin needling very superficially. Here one follows the divisions of the muscles. This applies to the upper and lower parts of the body. When one observes that the shen/spirit and color of the complexion return to normal, one should then remove the needles. In the winter one should acupuncture by deep insertion into the points. Here, as in severe illness, one can needle straight and deep, nearly to the depth of the bone. In less serious conditions, one can wiggle the needles from side to side and up and down, or insert additional needles slowly in points adjacent to the main point. These are the differing treatment methods for different seasonal needs.

"Since the qi of the human body flows in concert with that of heaven and earth, one must practice precisely according to where the qi is located. If in the spring one mistakenly needles the summer locations, the heart qi can be injured, causing the pulse to become irregular and weak. This will cause vulnerability to the pathogen and allow it to penetrate more deeply into the body, invading the bone and marrow and weakening the heart/fire. Since fire produces earth, this will manifest in symptoms such as lack of appetite and lethargy. In the spring if one mistakenly needles the autumn positions, causing injury to the lung qi, what will manifest are spasms in the tendons, and rebellious qi, such as cough and dyspnea. The pathogen will then be allowed to attack the lungs directly, resulting in severe cough, which can become chronic and even incurable. The liver qi is in turn injured, causing one to be easily startled. Once the lung qi is weakened, one becomes preoccupied with sadness and grief.

"In the spring if one mistakenly needles the winter position, the kidneys will be injured, allowing the pathogen to penetrate directly into the deep zang organs. This creates stagnation, distension, and fullness, with a grave prognosis. The liver qi will weaken and cause one to talk incessantly. In the summer if one mistakenly needles the spring position, the liver qi will be further weakened, causing weakness of the muscles and tendons. If in summer one needles the autumn position, injuring the lung qi, this will cause a loss of voice. Metal is unable to produce water and nourish the

kidneys. This will produce in one a fear of being arrested. In summer if
one needles the winter position, this will injure the kidney qi, draining the
jing. Now water cannot sufficiently produce wood. This causes the liver to
flare up in anger and rage. In the autumn, if one mistakenly needles the
spring position, this will injure the liver qi, causing blood to rise to the
head and leading to restlessness and emotional instability.

"In the spring, if one mistakenly needles the summer position, this
will injure the heart qi. Thus, the heartfire will be unable to produce the
earth. This will make one hypersomnic, with excessive dreams. In the autumn if one needles the winter position, this will drain the kidneys. The
kidneys can no longer store, and the blood and qi will scatter. Thus one
will feel chilled. In winter if one mistakenly needles the spring position,
this will injure the liver qi. The liver qi becomes deficient, and the hun
cannot be housed. Thus, one will be tired and lethargic and yet unable to
sleep. If one does sleep, one will have vivid dreams. In winter if one mistakenly needles the summer position, the heart qi will be disturbed. Thus the
qi of the pulses and vessels will become deflated and will allow the pathogen to attack, causing bi syndrome or arthritic conditions. In winter if one
mistakenly needles the autumn position, the lungs will be injured. Water
metabolism will be disrupted and one will be constantly thirsty. These sce-
narios demonstrate the importance of administering treatment in synchrony
with universal energy changes. Proper treatment will prevent conditions
from worsening, while attempting to restore normalcy.

"When acupuncture is applied to the chest and abdomen, one must
be extremely careful to avoid the organs. For example, if one punctures the
heart, the patient will die in less than thirty minutes. If one punctures the
spleen, the patient will die in five days. If one punctures the kidneys, the
patient will die in one week. If one punctures the lungs, the patient will
die in five days. If one punctures the diaphragm, the patient will not die
immediately but will suffer and not live longer than one year. It is important, therefore, to know the positions of the internal organs so that one
may avoid them. It is recommended, when working on the chest and abdomen, to first wrap the area with thick cotton cloth. Then needle through
the cloth. It is important to be cautious here with deep puncturing. It is
also important to quiet oneself, focus one's mind, and choose a tranquil
environment for the patient. The practitioner's qi should be connected and
in tune with the patient's. This helps one avoid accidents. When acupuncturing boils and suppurative conditions, one can use a method of punctur-

ing directly on the lesion and then shaking the needle, so as to drain the pus. When needling a point on a channel, however, do not shake the needle. These are the general principles of acupuncture."

Huang Di asked, "Can you tell me what happens when the qi is on the verge of collapse in the twelve meridians?"

Qi Bo answered, "When the taiyang/bladder and small intestine channel collapses, the patient will manifest opisthotonos, a stiffness of the back, convulsive spasms, paleness, and spontaneous sweating. Once the sweating stops, death will ensue. When the shaoyang/gallbladder and san-jiao channel collapses, the patient will become deaf and all the joints and bones will become loose and dislocated. The eyes will stare straight ahead and stop turning. In one and one-half days, death will ensue. At the time of death, the face will turn green, then white. When the yangming/stom-ach and large intestine channel collapses, the patient's face will become paralyzed. Delirium and a yellow face follow. Swelling and muscular spasms will occur along the yangming channels of the legs and arms. The muscles turn numb, then stiff, then immobile. When the shaoyin/kidney and heart channel collapses, the patient's face will turn black. The gums will recede and the teeth will blacken. The abdomen becomes distended and stagnant. Death will follow shortly. When the taiyin/spleen and lungs channel col-lapses, one will see abdominal distension, fullness and stagnation, difficulty breathing, sighing, burping, and vomiting. As one vomits, the qi rebels upward to the face, causing redness. However, if the qi does not rebel to the head, it will stagnate, causing the face to turn black. As this occurs, the texture of the face becomes dull and withered. Shortly after, death ensues. When the jueyin/liver and pericardium channel collapses, the patient feels feverish in the chest, dryness of the throat, has frequent urination, restless-ness, and irritability. Gradually, the tongue becomes stiff and unable to move. In men, the scrotum contracts. Immediately after, one shall die. These are the descriptions of what occurs when the qi of the twelve chan-nels collapses."

CHAPTER 17

—

THE METHODS OF
PULSE EXAMINATION

—

H UANG DI asked Qi Bo, "Can you explain the methods of pulse examination?"

Qi Bo answered, "The best time of day to examine the pulse is ping dan, the intersection between the yin and the yang times, about midnight. But realistically, early morning is a good time. This is comparable to the best basal body temperature time upon first arising. At this time one has not labored, the yin qi has not been disturbed, and the yang qi has not been dispersed. No food has been consumed, the energy in the channels and collaterals is not falsely excess, and the qi is flowing evenly. Qi and blood are not flowing recklessly at this time. At the same time as examining the pulse, one should observe the patient's spirit through the eyes, and the color of the complexion to determine the health of the zang fu organs. By utilizing these varied methods in combination, a physician can determine the life or death of the patient.

"The pulse is where the blood flows and congregates. The blood is mobilized by the qi. If we see a long pulse, it indicates that the qi is flowing smoothly. If we see a short pulse, it indicates that there is pathology at the qi level. If we see a rapid pulse, it indicates that the disease has attacked the heart. If we see a large pulse, it indicates that the pathogen is progressing. If the most superficial level of the pulse is strong and excess, it indicates that the qi is rebelling upward. If the deep position is excess and strong, it indicates that the qi is stagnant in the interior of the body. If the pulse is choppy, this means that the qi is collapsing. This is a pulse wherein one can feel the systolic but barely the diastolic. If the pulse is thready and small, this means that the qi is insufficient. If the pulse is irregular, this indicates heart pain. If the pulse emerges like a rushing spring, this means that the illness is worsening, with a poor prognosis. If initially the pulse is faint, but suddenly becomes wiry, this is a sign of death.

"If the face manifests redness, one must distinguish between a moist red and one that is without brightness. The normal color should be like silk cloth wrapping cinnabar. If the face is white, it should be lustrous, like goose feathers. It should not be like the color of salt. If the face is green, it should be like jade, not blue-green with a dark tinge to it. If the face is yellow, it should be like wrapping silk cloth over xiong huang/realgar, unlike the dirt of the Yellow River. If the face is black, it should be like black lacquered paint, unlike ashes in a grave. This means that if the five colors are expressed upon the face with the wrong qualities, the person will not live much longer. Healthy organs will manifest a healthy luster. Without this expression of the five colors, the jing/essence of the organs is departing and coming to the surface. These colors give the physician the basis for a prognosis. The lustrous colors indicate a better prognosis than the dull colors. However, even the lustrous colors must not be obvious. When obvious, even the healthy colors can indicate an extreme consequence.

"The eyes indicate the sufficiency of jing/essence. When the eyes degenerate in function, this indicates that the jing is exhausted.

"The five zang organs all have their responsibilities. If the abdomen is full, the qi of the zang organs is distended and there is dyspnea, usually induced by fear. The voice is turbid and not clear. This is unregulated middle jiao qi due to dampness. If the voice is feeble and repetitive, this is zheng sheng or unconscious speech. This means that the zheng qi is depleted. If the patient is restless and tossing and turning with delirium, this is zhan yu or delirious babbling. This is because the spirit is disturbed and disrupted. If the intestines and stomach cannot store the food and fluids, and diarrhea occurs, this indicates that the door to the house is not regulated. If there is incontinence the bladder cannot store and govern the turbid fluids. The above described disorders can be restored to normalcy if the five zang organs also restore their normal functioning. If they cannot do so, then the condition will worsen and eventually lead to death.

"Though the patient can live with the above diseases, if the diseases are not rectified the patient will eventually die. Thus, it can be said that uncontrolled bowel movements and incontinence are very serious.

"The five extraordinary palaces are the structural foundation for a strong, healthy body. The head is the palace of jing/essence. So, if one finds the head drooping, unable to rise, and finds the eyes sunken and without light, this indicates that the jing/essence and shen/spirit are about to collapse.

"The back is the palace for the chest. If the body is bowed like a humpback and the shoulders are drooping, this means that the qi of the chest is about to collapse. The lower back, or lumbosacral area, is the palace of the kidneys. If one loses mobility here, this means that the kidneys are about to collapse or degenerate. The knees are the palace of the tendons. So if one cannot bend or straighten them properly or needs to overcompensate in order to move, this means that the tendons are about to degenerate. The bones are the palace of the marrow. If one cannot stand for prolonged periods or walk with stability, this means that the bones are about to be exhausted. If the functions of the five palaces can be restored to normalcy, the person can be strengthened again and healed. If these five palaces cannot be restored, the illness shall progress and death will result."

Qi Bo continued, "There are four seasonal pulses. In the spring the pulse is naturally tense; in the summer the pulse is full; in the autumn it is floating; in the winter the pulse is sunken. But otherwise, when the pulse is large, the pathogen is excessive. When it is small, this means that the antipathogenic qi is deficient. In a condition of excess yang, the pulse should be big and floating. If it is small and thready, this means that the pathogenic qi is extremely excess. Contrarily, in the case of yin excess, where the pulse should be thready and small, if we observe a flooding and large pulse, this means that the antipathogenic qi is rapidly disintegrating. There is a term for this: guan ge, the yang cannot penetrate, the yin cannot expand. This indicates that the yin and the yang qi are stuck and are unable to assist one another."

Huang Di asked, "Can you explain to me the pulses of the four seasons? How is it that, through examination of the pulses, one can discover the location of the pathogen, know the progression of the pathogen, and understand whether the pathogen is on the surface or in the interior of the body? Can you please explain these factors to me in detail?"

Qi Bo answered, "The cycles of heaven and earth reflect in the constant changes in nature. Take the example of seasonal weather changes, from the warming trends of the spring, which give rise to the blazing heat of summer, which in turn changes into the coolness of the autumn and finally the severe cold of winter. Every organism in nature adapts and changes along with the seasonal cycles of germination in the spring, growth and development in the summer, maturity and harvest of the autumn, and storing or hibernating in the winter. The human pulse also corresponds to these changes. In the spring, the pulse will mirror nature and become slightly wiry or round; in the summer, it will enlarge and become flooding; in the fall, the pulse will float to the surface; in the winter, it will sink to the interior. From the beginning, the first day of winter, for forty-five days, the yang qi of nature gradually increases while the yin qi declines. From the first day of summer, for forty-five days, the yin qi begins to rise while the yang qi begins to decline. This is the natural law of yin and yang complementing each other; as one rises, the other descends. They thereby mirror the changes in the seasons.

"The pulses also follow this universal law of nature, corresponding to the changes of yin and yang energy. However, when the pulses fail to mirror the seasons, they have become pathological. By analyzing the pulses, we can determine the location of the illness. By then determining the excess or deficiency of the organs, we can foresee the progression. The key is to detect the subtle changes and differentiation of the pulses in order to know the future progression. Grasping the principles of the dynamics of yin and yang, understanding the cycles of the five elements, having the knowledge of the four seasonal energy factors, utilizing the principles of tonification and sedation at the precise moment and with the proper strength, using the appropriate timing of the seasons, are the essentials for efficient treatment. To do this, people and nature must form a union. In summary, the sound, the color of the complexion, and the pulses should all reflect the balance of yin and yang, of the five elements, and of the four seasonal changes of nature.

"When examining the pulse, there is a method one should follow. First, one must quiet one's mind and sharpen one's spirit. At the same time, one must know the normal pulses as they occur in the four seasons.

"In spring the pulse is slightly wiry, like the ripple or crest of a wave created by a fish swimming in a stream. The summer pulse is flooding and appears big at the skin level. This is more like the surging waves in the ocean. The autumn pulse is just beneath the skin, as if insects are preparing their homes for winter. The winter pulse is deep and to the bone, as if an animal were hibernating in a cave. When there is an imbalance in the body's interior, one should examine the pulse at the deepest level. But one must differentiate it from the normal pulse of winter. If there is illness of the superficial level, or exterior, one must compare the deep and superficial levels, thereby distinguishing from the normal spring pulse. This describes the six aspects of examining the pulse with regard to the four seasons and interior and exterior differentiation.''

Here Qi Bo made a digression to describe another diagnostic aid. "Dreams can also help us diagnose a person's illness. If one dreams of fearfully crossing a large body of water, this indicates an excess of yin. If one dreams of flames or fire, this indicates an excess of yang. If one dreams of mutual destruction between the subject and another person, this means both yin and yang are in excess. If one dreams of flying, there is an excess in the upper body. If one dreams of falling, there is an excess in the lower body. If one dreams of giving food to another, this means there is food retention. If one dreams of searching for food, there is emptiness in the middle jiao. If one is excessively angry in dreams, the liver is in excess. If one dreams of crying, the lungs are in excess. If one dreams of a gathering of crowds, this indicates short worms. If one dreams of fighting in a crowd, this indicates long worms. In these cases, grinding of the teeth and itchiness in the rectal area will also occur.''

Qi Bo continued, "When the heart pulse is rapid and full, this indicates that excess heat is exhausting the jin and ye/body fluids. Because the heart opens to the tongue, the tongue will be contracted and unable to speak. When the heart pulse is found to be slow and weak, this indicates that the pathogenic qi is gradually decreasing but that the jin and ye have not yet been restored. Once they have been restored, recovery will occur. When the lung pulse is rapid and full, this indicates that excess heat has injured the lung channel, causing blood to extravasate, as in the coughing up of blood. When the lung pulse is slow and weak, this indicates that the lung qi is unable to contain the jin ye. Spontaneous sweating will occur, and one should refrain from using diaphoresis. When the liver pulse is rapid and full, the face may often be greenish. If the face does not turn green, this indicates trauma and blood stagnation under the ribs. This can also cause dyspnea by obstructing lung qi. If the liver pulse is slow and weak, but the face manifests a moist, lustrous quality like water, one should suspect water retention deep within the body. This may be from abusive drinking habits due to thirst, causing the water to flood beyond the stomach and intestines.

"When the stomach pulse is rapid and full and the face is red, stomach fire is blazing. Since the stomach channel runs down the thigh, the patient may feel as if the femur is broken. If the stomach pulse is slow and weak, this means that the stomach qi is deficient and unable to perform the function of decomposing and ripening the food. The food is then retained, causing stagnation and pain. When the spleen pulse is rapid and full, and the face is yellowish, this usually indicates excess damp and heat, which obstruct the spleen's transformative process. When the spleen pulse is slow and weak, and the face is sallow, this indicates that the spleen yang is insufficient and unable to regulate the water. Water then flows downward and accumulates in the leg and foot area as edema. When the kidney pulse is rapid and full and the face is yellow with a red tinge, this means damp heat has injured the kidneys. Since the lower back is the palace of the kidneys, the lower back will be painful, as if broken. If the kidney pulse is slow and weak, this indicates that the jing and blood are depleted. Because the kidney is the source of prenatal essence, when jing and blood are depleted from the kidneys, it is very difficult to recover."

Huang Di asked, "When one detects a tense and rapid pulse in the heart area, what does this mean?"

Qi Bo replied, "It is xin shan, or heart hernia. When this occurs the lower abdomen bulges and there is a lump."

Huang Di asked, "How does this form?"

Qi Bo answered, "The heart provides fire and corresponds to the small intestine. In this case, cold has attacked the heart and transferred to its paired organ, where it coagulates and forms a lump."

Huang Di then asked, "When you feel the stomach pulse, what do you look for?"

Qi Bo answered, "If the stomach pulse is excess or full, there is a stagnation and one will find distension in the epigastrium. If the stomach pulse is weak, there is a deficiency of stomach qi and one is unable to process the food. This will result in diarrhea."

Huang Di asked, "When a pathogen invades the human body, what exactly is it that happens?"

Qi Bo answered, "When the wind carries a pathogen, it attacks the skin. One will then manifest fever and chills. If it is a heat pathogen, one will manifest an exhaustion of the middle jiao. It progresses into the yang-ming channel with signs of a big pulse, big fever, big sweat, and big thirst. When the qi rebels upward and disturbs the head, this may cause fainting or syncope. When the wind chronically attacks the stomach, chronic diarrhea will ensue. Also, when wind cold stagnates in the channels, a condition called li feng, wind cold residing in the channels, develops. This is leprosy. In conclusion, because of the ever-changing manifestations of pathogens, we can give only these examples. It is impossible to discuss them all."

Huang Di proceeded, "What about the many kinds of musculoskeletal problems, such as those of the tendons, bones, swelling, and boils? How are these brought about?"

Qi Bo answered, "Exposure to cold pathogens combined with wind is usually the cause."

Huang Di asked, "How does one treat these problems?"

Qi Bo answered, "These types of conditions usually come from abnormal changes in weather. One should follow the principles of yin and yang in dealing with these problems. Simply put, warm the cold, dry the damp, and cool the heat."

Huang Di asked, "Some illnesses come from actual disorders of the zang organs. How does one differentiate whether these are chronic conditions or acute?"

Qi Bo answered, "This is a good question. One merely has to examine the patient's pulse and complexion. For example, if the pulse is deficient or small but the complexion is still normal, this indicates an acute condition or new illness. But if the pulse is normal and the complexion has changed, this condition is chronic. If the pulse and complexion are both abnormal, this indicates a chronic condition. If the pulse and complexion are both normal, the condition is just beginning. If the kidney and liver pulses are deep and wiry and the complexion is dull and red, this usually indicates an acute, severe onset of illness that has caused damage and stagnation to the channels and blood. When this occurs, there will be generalized swelling in addition to the blood stagnation."

Qi Bo continued, "On each wrist there are three positions when a physician lays his index, middle, and ring fingers to detect subtle quality of pulse patterns. Cun is at the wrist, guan is on the styloid process of the radius, while the chi is proximal to the guan. All are located over the radial artery."

Qi Bo continued, "The two positions of the chi reflect the area below the ribs. These encompass the kidneys at the deep level and the abdomen at the superficial level. On the left guan position, the liver is reflected at the deep level, while the diaphragm manifests at the superficial level. The cun position of the left wrist shows the heart at the deep level and the pericardium at the superficial level. On the right wrist cun position, the lung reflects in the deep position while the chest shows on the superficial position. On the right guan, the stomach is at the deeper level, while the spleen is on the more superficial level. So we can say that the cun positions generally reflect the chest, the guan reflect from the epigastrium to the abdomen, the chi positions reflect the abdomen down to the feet."

Qi Bo then stated, "When the pulse is full and excessive, this means that the yin fluids are deficient and the yang is excessive. This refers to excess heat in the interior. When the pulse arrives quickly but leaves slowly, or the systolic is rapid and the diastolic recedes slowly, this indicates an excess in the upper jiao and a deficiency in the lower jiao/cavity. The qi has rebelled upward and can cause loss of consciousness. When the pulse is reversed, that is, the systolic is slow and the diastolic is rapid, this indicates deficiency in the upper jiao/cavity and excess in the lower jiao. It indicates an attack of wind that we call li feng, or leprosy. The yang qi is attacked first.

"If the pulse is deep, thready, and rapid, this indicates kidney yin deficiency with yang rising. If the pulse is deep, thready, rapid, and scattered, this indicates that the yin is insufficient and the exogenous factor has invaded, causing fever and chills. When the pulse is floating and dispersing, this indicates that the yin is severely depleted and the yang is floating on the surface. In this case, one would see vertigo, fainting, or unconsciousness. If the pulse is floating and quiet, this means that one will have fever. The pathogen will then be in one of the three foot yang channels. If the pulse is floating and reckless, this means that the pathogen is located in the three yang channels of the hand. If the pulse is thready and deep, this indicates that the condition is interior in nature and one may have joint pain. Here the pathogen is located in the three yin channels of the hand. If the pulse is thready, deep and quiet, this means that the pathogen is in the foot yin channels. If the pulse is rapid but with regular breaks, which we term regular irregular, the condition is of a yang nature. One will see diarrhea or pus and blood in the stools.

"Most varieties of excess pulses with choppy characteristics indicate that the pathogen has injured the yang level; however, the yang qi is still sufficient. If the pulse manifests as slippery, this means that the pathogen has invaded the yin level; however, the yin qi is still sufficient. When the yang qi is still sufficient, the body will become hot or feverish without sweating. If the yin qi is still sufficient, there will be chills and sweating. If the yin or yang qi is not severely damaged one will have chills without sweating. If one suspects that the pathogen is on the exterior, but the pulse is deep and not floating, this indicates that the condition is actually of an interior nature and possibly the epigastrium or abdomen has stagnation. Conversely, if symptoms and signs point to an interior condition, but the pulse is floating and not deep, this is actually an exterior condition. This will be a heat condition. If one suspects the condition is in the upper part of the body and the lower pulse is rather weak, one can say that there is an excess in the upper and a deficiency in the lower. The patient will manifest coldness and weakness in the lower back and legs. If the condition is suspected to be of the lower body and the lower pulse manifests excess, while the upper pulse shows deficiency, the yang is heavy and cannot rise, thus, one will suffer from head and neck pain."

Qi Bo concluded by saying, "What is a deep pulse? A deep pulse is where one must press all the way to the bone level to find it. This is because there is insufficiency of qi within the pulses and the flow of blood is weakened. In this case one may see a choppy pulse. A choppy and deep pulse is very deficient and indicates that the blood is not flowing freely. Here one will see back pain, stiffness of the entire body, and difficulty in gait and mobility."

CHAPTER 18

—

PULSE ANALYSIS

—

Huang Di asked, "What kind of pulse do you find in a normal person?"

Qi Bo answered, "The pulse of a normal, healthy individual will beat twice with each inhalation and twice with each exhalation. With one complete breath, there are four beats. Occasionally, it is normal to detect five beats per breath, depending on the patient's lung capacity.

"When palpating the pulse, one should feel it in reference to the patient's breath, if the patient is normal. However, if the pulse is more than five beats per patient's breath, this is abnormal. In this case, the physician should examine the pulse in reference to his or her own breathing. If there are only two beats per breath, there is a deficiency of qi. If there are three beats per breath, but the beats are rapid and the patient is irritable, and if the skin of the chi position is warm, this is febrile disease. If the skin is not warm and the pulse is slippery, this is a wind condition. If the pulse is choppy, this is a bi condition. If the pulse beats four or more times per exhalation, the condition is fatal. If the pulse does not arrive, this is also fatal, as are pulses that are intermittently rapid or slow.

"The source of a healthy pulse is the stomach. The pulse reflects stomach qi. If one detects the pulse readily, but there is insufficient stomach qi, this yields a poor prognosis.

"In the spring a wiry pulse is normal. But it should also display the moderate strength and gentle speed of the stomach qi. If the wiry quality dominates, the liver is unbalanced. When there is only a wiry quality and lacking stomach qi, the prognosis is poor. If the stomach qi exists in the pulse but there is also a floating quality, the patient will be diseased by autumn. If the floating pulse dominates, the disease will be acute and appear sooner. In the spring the liver should disseminate the qi of the five zang organs. The liver is also responsible for gathering the qi with which to nourish the tendons.

"In the summer the pulse should be like a flood but with the soft and gentle quality of the stomach qi. If the flooding quality dominates, this indicates trouble with the heart. If we detect only the flooding pulse, with no quality of stomach qi, death will ensue. When we encounter the pulse sinking like a stone during summer, this indicates that disease will come in the winter. If the sinking heavy pulse dominates, the condition will be acute.

"In late summer we should normally see a soft pulse possessing stomach qi. If the pulse is overly deficient and soft, with weak stomach qi, the spleen is diseased. If the pulse is intermittent with absence of stomach qi, the prognosis is poor. If the pulse is deep, sinking, and stonelike, but also weak, the illness will manifest quickly. In late summer the qi of the five zang organs converges in the spleen. This allows the spleen to nourish the flesh and muscles. If in autumn we have a floating hairlike pulse with little stomach qi, the lung is diseased. If there is no stomach qi, death will ensue. When a floating pulse is combined with a wiry quality, one will become ill in the spring. If the wiry quality dominates, one will become ill immediately. In the autumn the five zang qi converge at the lungs. This aids the lungs in dispersing and transporting the ying/nutritive and wei/defensive qi throughout the body. In the winter, if the deep, stony pulse is unaccompanied by adequate stomach qi, the kidneys are diseased. If there is an absolute absence of stomach qi, the prognosis is poor. If a sinking pulse combines with a flooding pulse, illness will come the following summer. If the flooding quality dominates, one will become ill immediately. In the winter, the qi of the five zang organs is stored in the kidneys, allowing the kidneys to harbor the bone marrow.

"The stomach channel has a large collateral called shu li. Its path leads from the stomach across the diaphragm and connects to the lungs. One can feel its pulsation under the left breast. This is the root of the pulse qi. If it is pulsating rapidly and strong, but skips a beat, the disease is at shangzhong (REN17) in the chest. If the pulse is choppy and displaced sideways, this indicates stagnation. If the physician cannot feel this pulse qi at all, the patient will die; and if one can observe the pulsation through the clothing, the root qi is escaping.

"When palpating the radial pulse, one must understand the proper positioning of the finger on the cun pulse. If the pulse here is short, the yang qi is deficient, and one will have headaches. If the pulse is long, the yin is deficient and one will have foot or heel pain. If the pulse here is hurried and full, the yang is in excess; there will then be pain in the scapula. If the pulse is hard and full, there is excess yin and the condition is internal. If the pulse is floating and full, the condition is yang and located at the surface. If the pulse is sinking and frail, and one can palpate it only deeply, the condition is internal; this is usually due to heat or cold stagnation in the abdomen, causing a mass. If the pulse is sinking and has a tendency to move across the width of the wrist, the yin qi is coagulating and there is stagnation under the ribs; there may also be abdominal pain. If the pulse is sinking and hurried, there is simultaneous cold and heat."

Qi Bo continued, "Generally speaking, without regard to a particular position, when the pulse is small, frail, and choppy, this indicates deficient and chronic conditions. If the pulse is full, slippery, and hard, the condition is yang and on the outside. If the pulse is small, full, and hard, the condition is yin and internal. If the pulse is floating, slippery, and rapid, the condition is excess and acute. If the pulse is wiry and rapid, it is a liver pulse. There may be hernia or stagnation in the lower abdomen. If the pulse is very slippery, this is a yang condition and wind is involved. If the pulse is choppy, the condition is yin and involves bi syndrome or arthritic conditions. If the pulse is slow and slippery, it is a spleen condition. This indicates that heat is attacking the middle jiao. If the pulse is full and tight, yin and yang are struggling, and one will likely have abdominal distension. If the pulse corresponds to the manifestation of the illness, the condition is easily cured. If this is not so, the case is difficult. If the pulse is in accordance with the four seasons, there is no danger. If the pulse is opposite to the appropriate season and does not follow the normal course of transmission, the condition is dangerous.

"If the arm has many visible veins, the indication is blood deficiency or blood loss. If the pulse in the chi position at the radial artery by the wrist is slow, but the overall pulse is choppy, qi and blood are deficient and the patient will tend to be hypersomnic. If the pulse is full, there is fire within the body; there may be excess bleeding. If there is choppiness in the chi position, but the overall pulse is slippery, yang qi is excessive within and there will be profuse sweating. If the skin over the chi position is cool and the pulse is thin, coldness is within and one may have diarrhea. If the pulse is large and thick and the skin over the chi position is warm, there is heat in the middle. If the zhen zang mai—or pulse condition representing the decaying of visceral energy, thus a decaying liver pulse—appears, one will die by gen xin day of the energy almanac. If the decaying pulse of the heart appears, one will die by ren kui day. If the decaying pulse of the spleen appears, one will die by jia yi day. If the decaying pulse of the lung appears, one will die by bing ding day. If the decaying pulse of the kidney appears, one will die by wu ji day. The knowledge of this is based on an energetic almanac that I shall discuss later. These dates I mentioned simply correspond to the organ systems whereby astronomy is observed to exert influence.

"If the carotid pulse in the neck is rapid and accompanied by dyspnea and cough, this is a condition involving water imbalance. If the eyes are swollen and protruding, it is also a water condition. If there is dark yellow urine with a reddish tinge, accompanied by hypersomnia, jaundice is possible. Yellow sclera also indicate jaundice; hunger after eating is a type of jaundice, too. A swollen face indicates water and wind. Foot and ankle swelling is water retention.

"If in women the hand shaoyin or the heart pulse is prominent, pregnancy is indicated. Pulses that are opposite to their appropriate seasons are known as rebellious. The pulse in a wind-heat condition should be floating, rapid, and irritable. If instead it is sinking and quiet, the condition is an example of a rebellious pulse. In a case of diarrhea and bleeding, the pulse should be empty; if instead it is full, this is rebellious. If a condition is internal and excess but the pulse is empty, this is also a rebellious pulse. If the condition is external but the pulse is hard and choppy, this, too, is a rebellious pulse. Conditions displaying rebellious pulses are difficult to treat.

"The source of vitality is the diet. If one stops eating or drinking, one will die. Without food or liquid, stomach qi will not be evident in the pulses. The lack of stomach qi in the pulses usually indicates death. What is meant by no stomach qi? The physician feels only the decaying pulse, without the gentle strength of the stomach qi. For example, the decaying pulse of the liver is slightly wiry, without any strength. The decaying pulse of the kidney should be slightly sinking, not truly sinking.

"A taiyang condition should have a long and flooding pulse; a shaoyang condition should display an irregular, intermittently rapid and slow or intermittently long and short pulse; a yangming condition should display a floating, large, and short pulse.

"Normally, the pulse of the heart is like a strand of pearls; it flows continuously beneath the fingertips. If the pearls arrive rapidly, without rhythm, and seem to veer off the track, the indication is pathology of the heart. If the pulse wave is curved in the beginning and straight in the end, and there is no softness, this is called the death pulse of the heart.

"The normal lung pulse is light, floating, and soft; neither rushed nor slow. It is like a leaf falling from a tree. If the pulse does not float back and forth with the downward motion of the leaf, it is considered a pathologic pulse of the lung. If the pulse wave feels like an object floating on the surface of water and has no root, this is the death pulse of the lung.

"The normal liver pulse feels like the end of a long bamboo stick and is springy. If it feels slippery and full, like the hard bamboo pole, this is a pathologic liver pulse. If it appears as a new bow, taut and tense, this is the death pulse of the liver.

"The normal spleen pulse is soft, harmonious, and rhythmic, like the feet of a chicken as they touch the ground while walking. If the pulse is full and rapid, like the chicken lifting its feet, this is a pathologic pulse of the spleen. If the pulse wave appears like the beak or claws of a bird, sharp and hard, or like a roof leaking randomly, or water flowing downstream, never to return, this is the death pulse of the spleen.

"The normal kidney pulse has a round, smooth, slippery quality; it has a slight tendency to sink. If the pulse wave appears to be a large climbing vine, hard and not smooth or round, the indication is imbalance of the kidneys. If the pulse appears to be two people fighting over something, as in a tug of war, unpredictable, hard, and erratic, with tension, as hard as a marble, this is the death pulse of the kidney."

CHAPTER 19

SEASONAL VARIATIONS AND ABNORMALITIES IN PULSES

Huang Di asked, "Can you describe the normal and the abnormal pulses of each season?"

Qi Bo replied, "In spring the pulse should be slightly wiry. Its quality is soft, light, slightly hollow, and slippery, straight but long. The summer pulse should be like a flood. It corresponds to the heart. As it arrives it is full, and as it leaves it becomes lighter. The autumn pulse should float slightly. As it arrives it is light and not strong; as it leaves it is quick and disperses. The winter pulse should be heavy like a stone. As it arrives it sinks and grabs the finger.

"If during these seasons the pulse does not correspond to the above, a pathology is in evidence. For example, if the spring pulse feels strong and full; if the summer pulse is strong and powerful coming and going; if the autumn pulse is floating and soft but hard at the middle level and hollow at the superficial and deep levels; if the winter pulse feels hard and springy like a slingshot—these are all excess conditions primarily affecting the exterior of the body. If the spring pulse is minute; if the summer pulse is not strong coming but is strong going; if the autumn pulse is soft, floating and minute; if the winter pulse is empty and rapid—these are all deficient conditions primarily affecting the interior.

"If in the spring one manifests an excessive pulse, one will have poor memory, dizziness, vertigo. If one has a deficient pulse in the spring, one will have chest pains that pierce through to the back. The hypochondriac area will be full and distended. If one has an excess pulse in the summer, one will manifest fever and pain in the epidermis. Boils, carbuncles, and skin lesions will form. If one has a deficient pulse in summer, one will have irritability, anxiety, palpitations, and excessive salivating, resulting in collapse of the yang qi in the lower body. This would result in diarrhea, spermatorrhea, and so forth. If one has an excess pulse in the autumn, one will have dyspnea and back pain, fullness and discomfort in the trunk. A deficient autumn pulse will be accompanied by shortness of breath, asthma, cough, and coughing up blood. There will be breath sounds from the throat. An excess pulse in the winter will be accompanied by lack of energy, focus, and concentration, weakness in body and limbs, pain in the bones and vertebrae, shallow breath, a feeble voice, and a dislike of speaking. When the winter pulse is deficient, one will feel an empty and hollow feeling in the heart area, tremendous hunger, gurgling in the abdomen, coldness below the ribs as if sitting in water, vertebrae pain, a distended lower abdomen, and dysuria.

"The normal pulse of late summer, corresponding to the earth element, is not obvious. When this pulse is excess, it feels like water dispersing in all directions. This indicates that the illness is on the exterior. One will manifest immobility of the extremities. When this pulse is deficient, it feels sharp and hard like the beak of a bird pecking. This means that the illness is in the middle, neither inside or outside. One will experience congestion and stoppage of all nine orifices. The body feels heavy and the tongue is stiff."

Qi Bo went on, "There is also a pattern of disease we can call the abnormal transmission of pathogenic qi. This specifically refers to cases of excess. In this abnormal sequence, the disease that is manifesting in its host organ was transmitted from the son of that element. For example, pathogenic qi of the heart was transmitted from the son of fire, the spleen, or earth. Now that the heart is excess, it transfers its pathogenic qi to the element that it controls, metal or lungs. Once the lungs are pathogenic, their qi is transmitted to the element that metal controls, which is wood, or liver. Because the element that wood controls, the earth, is already excess, the wood then insults its mother, the water or kidneys. When the sequence reaches this point, where all five zang organs have been affected, death is imminent." [Another way of speaking about this condition is to say that heart disease, in the form of atherosclerosis, may be generated by cholesterol from spleen dampness. The heart disease may cause congestive or pulmonary edema, which causes difficulty breathing. That in turn causes backup into the liver in the form of portal hypertension. This high pressure then leads to failure of the kidneys.]

"This pattern of transmission can apply to all the zang organs. Therefore, if the spleen is the host organ, we say that its pathogenic qi came from the son, or lungs. The spleen then passes the disease to the kidneys, the kidneys to the heart, and finally the heart to the liver, whereupon death occurs. If the lungs are the host, the pathogenic qi arose from their son, or kidneys. From the lungs, the disease progresses to the liver, then spleen, and last the heart, whereupon death transpires. Should the kidneys be the host, the pathogenic qi initially transmits from the son or liver. The sequence in this case is then to the heart, the lungs, culminating in the spleen. There are many clinical examples for each of these sequences.

"In summary, we can say that when disease is about to become grave, it must originate with the son and subsequently be passed on to the element the host organ controls. We could label this the rebellious, abnormal transformation cycle, and it has definite application in practice with grave diseases. We can predict the time of death by having knowledge of the biorhythm of the body. For example, the time period around midnight corresponds to the liver or wood element, early morning to the lung or metal element, near noon the heart or fire element, afternoon the spleen or earth element, and before midnight the kidney or water element. By understanding this abnormal sequence, we can see where to intercede in order to interrupt the disease cycle and thereby prevent death."

Huang Di answered, "So the five zang organs are interconnected, intercommunicating, and interdependent. And the progression and transformation of pathogenic factors have their specific order. Therefore, when each of the five zang organs becomes diseased, it often passes evil qi to the element it controls. In such cases, if one does not treat in a timely fashion, the patient can live at most three to six months, or at the least, three to six days. Once the disease progresses through all five zang organs in this abnormal way, death will follow. If one is able to differentiate the three different yang channels, one can know what from which channel the disease originated. If one is able to differentiate the three yin channels, one can then know the prognosis and date of death."

Qi Bo went on to say, "Pathogenic wind heads the six pathogenic factors. It is often called the leader of the rebellion. When wind cold invades, it causes one's body hair to be erect and the pores to close. Thus it brings on fever, and one should use diaphoretic methods to induce sweating and eliminate the pathogen. When wind cold invades the channels and collaterals, causing numbness, paralysis, or stiffness and pain, one can use heat packs, moxibustion, and acupuncture to disperse it. If the pathogen is not caught in time, it will transfer into the lungs and cause lung bi, or lung obstruction, leading to cough and dyspnea. If the treatment is not effective or properly applied, the pathogen will go from the lung to the liver. This will cause liver bi, or an obstruction of the liver. One will manifest hypochondriac pain and vomiting. Here, one can use massage or acupuncture. If these are still ineffective, the pathogen will transfer from the liver to the spleen. This will cause spleen wind, manifesting in jaundice, a burning sensation of the abdomen, restlessness, and scanty, dark urination. One can apply massage, herbs, or baths. If these are still ineffective, the disease will transfer from the spleen to the kidneys. This is called shan jia, or herniated mass. In this case the lower abdomen will have burning, pain, and distension. The urine will be white and turbid. This is also known as gu zhang or abdominal tympanites due to parasitic infection. One should utilize massage and herbs. If the problem is still unalleviated, the transmission is now from the kidneys to the heart. This will cause spasms and contractures of the limbs. This is called chi bing or spastic tendons. Moxibustion and herbs are indicated here. If treatment is still not effective, within ten days the patient shall die. However, if the pathogen passes from the kidney to the heart and then back to the lungs, causing chills and fever, the patient will die within three days. This is the general order of disease passage within the five-element scheme.

"An example of this would be a cold that progresses to bronchitis or pneumonia, producing water retention in the lungs. Blood then accumulates in the liver, which in turn backs up to the spleen and stomach. This is earth deficient, water overflooding, fire weakening, heart failing, finally causing aggravation of the original problem."

Qi Bo continued, "Illness of sudden onset may not necessarily follow the creative cycle, particularly emotional disorders. Worry, fear, grief, overexcitability, and rage, because they often do not follow the creative cycle, may result in a more severe disorder. Extremes of excitability injure the heart. When the heart is deficient, the kidney energy overcontrols. In cases of rage, the liver is in excess and invades the spleen. Grief causes the lung to overcontrol the liver. Fear weakens the kidneys and causes the spleen to overcontrol the kidneys. In excessive sadness, the lung qi becomes deficient, allowing the heart to dominate. These are illnesses, induced by emotional extremes, that do not follow the typical creative cycle but rather follow the control pattern. In ancient times there was a saying that although there are only five elemental illnesses, there are twenty-five variations.

"When the larger bones grow hollow and become brittle, when the major muscles atrophy, when the chest is full with difficulty breathing, one can expect the patient to die within six months. In this case one should palpate the pulse of the lungs to detect the true qi that remains. This enables one to predict the time of death. In addition to the above-mentioned signs, if one manifests pain in the chest radiating to the shoulder, this can indicate that the patient may pass away within one month. In this case, one would palpate for the decaying heart pulse. In addition, if a patient manifests fever and emaciation of the entire body, we palpate the spleen pulse to look for the decaying pulse of the spleen. In this condition, death may follow within ten days. Separately, when we also see degeneration of the bones and sinking of the flesh, where the marrow is depleting and movements are senile, if we cannot detect the decaying kidney pulse, the patient will survive up to one year. If the decaying kidney pulse is present then death shall ensue shortly. If there is abdominal pain and fullness of the epigastrium, and if in addition there is pain in the upper shoulders, fever, if the eyes are sunken and the vision is blurry, or if blindness occurs, we look for the presence of the decaying liver pulse. Sudden death may occur here. The patient who retains his or her eyesight will live until blindness occurs. If a case involves onset of illness with an exterior factor, the qi flow of the five zang organs suddenly becomes stagnant and permanently blocked, such as in traumatic injuries, including falling from a great height or drowning, here we cannot predict the time of death. However, if the pulse becomes faint, or one cannot properly detect it, or if the pulse is rapid for a short period, though physically the patient is not disfigured, death may still result.

"Perhaps we should define the decaying zang pulses. The decaying liver pulse, when arriving, feels as if one is pressing against the blade of a knife, or is as taut as if pressing on a stringed instrument. The face will also be green, pale, or dull in nature, and the body hair is withered and sloughing off. This pulse means death. The decaying pulse of the heart is short, round, and solid like the pearl barley seed. The complexion is dark, red, and dull. If the body hair is withered and sloughs off, this means death, too. The decaying pulse of the lungs is as light as a feather touching one's skin. The face is pale, red, and dull. Again the body hair is withered and sloughed off. This points to death as well. The decaying pulse of the kidneys is hard as a marble, but frail, as if a rope is on the verge of breaking. The face is yellowish, dull, or black, and the body hair is withered and sloughed off. This points to death. The decaying pulse of the spleen is irregular and weak; there is a dull yellowish-green complexion, and withered, sloughing-off body hair. All indicate death. When one encounters these five decaying pulses, death is always indicated."

Huang Di asked, "What is the mechanism behind the appearance of the decaying pulses, which all lead to death?"

Qi Bo answered, "The nutrients of the five zang organs are all derived from the stomach. The stomach is therefore considered the root of the five zang. The qi of the five zang cannot be transported to the radial pulse posiitons without the transportive function of the stomach along with its qi. When an illness is very grave, it affects the stomach qi and therefore prevents the stomach qi as well as the normal zang qi from reaching the radial pulse by the wrist. The only pulse appears is the pulse of the zang that has been overcome by the pathogen. This pulse is the decaying pulse of that zang organ, and when detected, death will follow."

Huang Di said, "In treatment, we should diagnose the patient's excess and deficiency, the health of the qi, the colors and glow of the complexion, and the strength and deficiency of the pulses. In this way we are able to differentiate chronic from acute illness. When the manifestations of the body and the qi correspond, this means the condition is treatable. When the facial complexion and color have luster, this is also a sign of a curable condition. When the pulse corresponds to the four seasons, the condition is easily treatable. When the pulse arrives weak but is smooth and regular, the stomach qi is intact and the condition is curable. However, when the physiology and qi do not correspond, the case is difficult. When the face is dull and sallow, the case is difficult. When the pulse is excessive and hard, the illness will worsen. When the pulse does not correspond to the four seasons, and is directly opposite, the condition is incurable. In these cases, we shall inform the patient and family members accordingly.

"What does it mean to say that the pulse is opposite? In the spring the pulse is that of the lungs; in the summer the pulse is that of the kidneys; in the autumn the pulse is that of the heart; in the winter the pulse is that of the spleen. A suspended pulse without root and a pulse that is so deep and choppy that it does not rise are both pulses that oppose the four seasons. In the spring or summer, if one sees a deep pulse, or if in the autumn or winter, one sees a floating pulse, these are also considered opposing the four seasons. In febrile disease or heat conditions, the pulse should be large and flooding. If it is small and quiet instead, this is an opposing pulse. In dysentery or diarrhea, the pulse should be small or thready. If it is large, this is an opposing condition. In the case of shock due to loss of fluids, dehydration, or extravasation, one should detect a deficient pulse. If there is an excess pulse instead, this is considered opposing, too. When the illness is clearly internal but the pulse is excess and hard, or when the illness is external and we find the pulse not external or hard, these, like the above-mentioned, are difficult to treat."

Huang Di added, "I have heard that by gauging the nature of excess and deficiency, one can render an accurate prognosis."

Qi Bo answered, "When there are five excesses of five deficiencies to the extreme, one may succumb. The heart dominates the vessels. When the pulse is excess, the heart has been invaded by excess pathogens. The lungs govern the skin. When the skin is hot, the lungs have been invaded by excess pathogens. The spleen governs the abdomen. When the abdomen is distended, the spleen has been invaded by excess pathogens. The kidneys oversee the lower orifices: urination and defecation. When these are blocked, the kidney has been invaded by excessive pathogens. The liver opens to the eyes. When there is blurriness and difficulty with vision, the liver has been invaded by excessive pathogens. These are considered to be the five excesses.

"When the pulse is thready, the heart qi is deficient. When there are chills of the skin, the lung qi is deficient. When there is a lack of mobility and strength, the liver qi is deficient. When there is incontinence of bowels and urine, the kidney qi is deficient. When one is unable to eat or drink, the spleen qi is deficient. These are the five deficiencies."

Huang Di inquired, "In the five excesses and the five deficiencies there have been recoveries. Why is that?"

Qi Bo answered, "If a patient can still eat porridge, the stomach qi is still intact. If diarrhea stops, that patient can still recover. If fever without sweating turns to fever with sweating, and if the urine and bowel were stuck but are now open, though the condition is excess, the patient can recover. Therefore, in deficient conditions, one can survive as long as the stomach qi is intact; in excess conditions, as long as the openings—pores, bowels, urine—remain open, the pathogen can be eliminated and the patient will recover. That is the mechanism that belies the rectification of the five excesses and the five deficiencies."

CHAPTER 20

—

DETERMINING LIFE AND DEATH

—

H UANG DI said, "In the past I have inquired about the knowledge of the nine needles. After your profound teachings, I finally understood the essence of this. I have taught it to my sons so it may be passed on and not forgotten. They know to pass on these secrets only with the utmost care and caution. I would now like to know the relationship of this information to the cosmos, to the seasonal correspondences, and how the human being fits into this natural law."

Qi Bo answered, "You have asked a very good question. This hinges on the esoteric understanding of the workings of the universe."

Huang Di said, "I would like to know how to utilize this knowledge to determine human life and death."

Qi Bo stated, "The science of cosmology as developed by the Taoist utilizes numerology, beginning with the number one and ending with the number nine. Odd numbers represent yang and heaven, while even numbers present yin and earth. The human being resides between heaven and earth and is represented by the number three. Heaven, earth, and the human being unite as three. Three generations of this three are nine.

"In the human being we discuss the three areas of the body. Within each area there are three locations where the pulses can be found, which we use to determine whether a patient will survive or die."

Huang Di asked, "Please tell me what these three areas are."

Qi Bo replied, "The human being consists of a lower, a middle, and an upper area. Within each there are three pulses, which represent heaven, earth, and the human being. These need to be revealed by an accomplished teacher so that one may accurately palpate them. In the upper area, heaven is represented at the ends of the eyebrows; earth is located in the cheeks; the human being is located in front of the ears. In the middle area, heaven is represented in the arteries of the hand taiyin; earth is represented in the arteries of the hand yangming/large intestine; the human being is represented in the arteries of the hand shaoyin/heart. In the lower area, heaven is represented by the arteries of the foot jueyin/liver; earth is represented by the arteries of the food shaoyin; the human being is represented by the arteries of the foot taiyin.

"It is also said that in the lower area, the heaven position can detect the qi of the liver; the earth position can detect the qi of the kidney; and the human position can detect the qi of the spleen and stomach."

Huang Di asked, "Please tell me about the middle area."

Qi Bo replied, "Within the middle area, in the heaven position one can detect the lung qi; in the earth position one can detect the qi of the chest; in the human position one can detect the qi of the heart."

Huang Di asked, "Please tell me about the upper area."

Qi Bo answered, "In the upper area, the heaven position detects the qi of the head; the earth position detects the qi of the mouth and teeth; the human position detects the qi of the ear and eyes. Within the human being, there are the lungs, liver, heart, spleen, and kidneys (the five zang organs), and the bladder, stomach, large intestine, and small intestine (the four fu/essential organs). The five zang are called the five spirit zang, and the four fu are called the four hollow zang. This combines to make nine zang, which correspond to the nine pulses of the human being and the nine continents of earth. If the five zang become diseased, one will see disintegration of the spirit, leading to death."

Huang Di asked, "What are the diagnostic techniques and procedures?"

Qi Bo answered, "One must first visually evaluate the patient's physical shape to understand the relative strength of the zheng qi or good qi and pathogens. If it is excessive with pathogen, one must sedate; if deficient, one must tonify. When one sedates, the initial work is to eliminate the stagnation in the blood vessels. Next, one regulates and tonifies qi and blood when they are deficient. Regardless of the type of illness, one must first regulate and balance the flow of qi and blood."

Huang Di asked, "How do you determine life and death?"

Qi Bo answered, "When the physical signs are excessive but the pulse is thin, and there is rapid dyspnea, shortness of breath, and difficulty breathing, the condition is serious. If the patient is deficient, and the outward appearance is skinny, but the pulse is full and large, death is usually indicated. Generally, when the outward appearance and the pulse correspond, there is hope for a cure. When the outward appearance and the pulse do not correspond, death is indicated. If the pulses of the upper and lower, and from left to right, do not match, then the problem is severe. If the difference is great, the indication is death. If the pulses in the middle area of the body are balanced and even, but the other areas are disharmonious, the indication is also death. If the pulses in the middle area are deficient and do not correspond to the pulses of the other areas, this also indicates death. If the qi is depleted to the point where the eye sinks into its socket, this also denotes death."

Huang Di asked, "How would one know where the illness is located?"

Qi Bo answered, "When you palpate the nine pulses, you will find where deficient and small pulses, large and full pulses, rapid and slow pulses, and floating and sinking pulses are located. These indicate the pathogen and its location. For example, with the left hand, press the patient's left leg on the medial side of the leg five cun above the ankle, then gently percuss the inside of the left ankle with your right hand for vibration to travel to the left hand. If you feel the vibration in your left hand rhythmically, this is normal. If the vibration detected is chaotic and uncorresponding, this is abnormal. If the vibration is slow and mild, illness is also indicated. If percussion is hard and there is no vibration felt, death may be imminent. When the muscle of the whole body emaciates to the point where one cannot walk, this too is a sign of death. In the middle area, if the pulse is intermittently slow and fast, this also means death. If the pulse is choppy and flooding, the pathogen is in the luo channels and the illness will manifest superficially.

"The nine pulses should be in concert to denote health. If two pulses are out of alignment, the problem is serious. If three pulses are divergent, the illness is very dangerous. When one attempts to diagnose pathogens within the organs, in order to detect either the time of death or of healing, one must understand the normal pulses. Then one can differentiate the true zang pulses and grasp the time of healing or death. For example, when the qi of the foot taiyang/bladder channel is exhausted, the feet cannot bend. When one dies, one will exhibit opisthotonos."

Huang Di said, "Winter is considered yin and summer is considered yang. How do the pulses correspond?"

Qi Bo answered, "If the nine pulses are all deep, thready, and faint, we consider them yin. This is similar to winter. If death occurs, it will be in the middle of the night. If the pulses are excess, irritable, and rapid, we consider them yang. This is like summer. Death will occur in the middle of the day. If there is a battle between hot and cold, one will die at the intersection of yin and yang, about one in the morning. In febrile disease, one will die at the hottest time of day, usually at noon. In wind conditions, one will die in the late afternoon, when yang is depleted. In water conditions one will die at the extreme of yin, the middle of the night. When the pulse manifests as intermittently rapid and slow, the spleen qi is dying. One will then pass away at chen, wu, chou, wei times—midnight, noon, and the twilight hours. If a patient develops paralysis, even if the nine pulses are in concert, it is grave and difficult to cure.

"If the nine pulses are in concert in shape despite an unhealthy quality of thin or small, large or full, rapid or slow, floating or sinking, this does not mean death. A condition caused by wind or menstrual problems or chronic conditions may display similar pulse qualities. Similarly, if the nine pulses are in concert but have an underlying frailty, indicating exhaustion of stomach qi, death is indicated. Death here will be preceded by vomiting. It is imperative that a doctor must be thorough in taking the medical history, investigating the current manifestations, and palpating and examining all pulses carefully. If the pulses flow easily and freely, the patient is generally safe; if the pulses are choppy, hesitant, or slow, disease is indicated. If the pulse fails, this means death. In paralysis where the muscles are wasting, death will soon follow."

Huang Di asked, "How do we proceed with treatable conditions?"

Qi Bo answered, "If the pathogen is located in the channel, acupuncture the channel. If the pathogen is in the small collaterals, bleed them. If the pathogen is in the blood and causes pain, treat both the channels and the collaterals. If the pathogen stagnates in the large collaterals of the right side, treat the left side, and vice versa. If the pathogen lingers stubbornly for a long period of time, treat the webs of the hands and feet, and the joints. Upon examining the pulses, if one distinguishes an excess of the upper and a deficiency of the lower, one must locate the stagnation. Then go to the source of the stagnation and bleed, in order to promote the qi flow. If a patient manifests opisthotonos, the eyes are rolling upward, the qi in the taiyang channel has been depleted. If the eyes are turned up but do not quiver, the qi in the taiyang channel is exhausted, and death is imminent. The indications I have discussed are the keys to determining life and death. You must pay utmost attention to them."

CHAPTER 21

—

MERIDIAN PATHOLOGY AND CORRESPONDING PULSE SIGNS

—

H UANG DI asked, "Do the qi and blood flowing within the channels and collaterals change according to the relative activity of a person's excesses and deficiencies?"

Qi Bo answered, "Yes. The qi and blood in the body are affected by the various movements of the person throughout the day. This includes the emotions of rage, fear, too much thinking, sadness, and joy. For example, when one stays up too late at night and is active, the kidney qi becomes depleted. This creates a condition of deficiency, with dyspnea or shortness of breath. Many people think the cause of this is the cold air, but it is actually due to depletion of the kidneys during the night. If one is attacked by exogenous factors during this time, the lungs will be injured. Or if one suffers fright falling from great height, shortness of breath and dyspnea would manifest as a result of the liver qi being affected, particularly when the ligament and tendons were sprained or strained, causing blood to congeal. If the liver qi becomes reckless as a result, the spleen will also be injured. Similarly, when one is frightened, the spirit scatters. Because the lungs gather the qi, dyspnea and shortness of breath will result from this as well. If the qi of the lungs becomes reckless, the heart will be injured. Another example would be if one tries to cross a stream but falls in. The water energy is connected to the kidneys, so this falling would result in shortness of breath and dyspnea too. Under all these circumstances, one who is strong and able will recover. If one is frail, the qi and blood will stagnate and illness will result. Therefore, as part of one's ability to diagnose correctly, one must be able to observe keenly the constitutional propensity of the patient, and the physical presentation of the skin, bones, flesh, and muscles."

Qi Bo continued, "One sweats from the stomach after one eats; one sweats from the heart after being startled; one sweats from the kidneys as a result of physical overstrain or from traveling long distances under a heavy load; one sweats from the spleen when one uses one's muscles; one sweats from the liver when one is running fearfully. Within the context of the yin/yang changes of the four seasons, the etiology of disease is often determined by one's constitution and expenditure, one's diet, activity level, and emotional tendencies."

"When food enters the stomach, it is digested and transformed. The heavier food essence is transported to the liver, nourishing the entire body's tendomuscular channels. Then the refined, substantial portion of the food essence is transported to the heart, through the blood vessels, channels, and collaterals, then it converges at the lungs, whereby the lungs dispense it to the hundred channels of the entire body and finally to the skin and body hair. From there it combines with the qi of the channels and is transported to the other four zang organs, where the essence is stored. The distribution of this essence must be even and effective. In this way its abundance can be detected at the radial pulse. This is also how one can determine the prognosis of the patient.

"Fluid enters the stomach. It is then extracted as a fluid essence, which is processed by the spleen. The spleen then separates the pure from the turbid. Within the pure, there are the jin and ye, which are transported to the lungs. The lungs, in their function of regulating water passages, distribute the purified fluids to the entire body via channels and collaterals and finally to the five zang, and eventually the turbid and waste fluid is transported to the bladder. The metabolism of food and fluids follows a certain order of the seasons and is affected by the balance of yin and yang and the proper functions of the zang fu.

"When the taiyang channel becomes excess, conditions of dyspnea, rebellious qi, and contractures occur. They indicate an insufficiency of yin and an excess of yang. One should sedate both the exterior and interior, using acupuncture points shugu (B65) on the foot taiyang and the taixi (K3) on the foot shaoyin channels. When the yangming channel is excess, the taiyang and shaoyang channels are also excessive. This is a condition of tremendous abundance of yang. One should sedate acupuncture points xian gu (ST43) on the foot yangming and tonify tai bai (SP3) on the foot taiyin points. When the shaoyang channel is in excess, one may pass out. The diagnosis can be confirmed with the pulse in the shaoyang position. The remedy is acupuncturing points zhuling qi (G41) on the foot shaoyang channel. When the taiyin channel is disturbed and the taiyin pulse is abnormally distinct, one should take care to rule out a decaying zang pulse. If the qi of the five zang organs has been depleted and the stomach qi is correspondingly out of balance, this is a case of taiyin being excess. In this case, one should tonify by acupuncturing xiangu (ST43) on the foot yangming channel, and sedate by acupuncturing taibai (SP3) on the foot taiyin channel. In shaoyin heat excess, the deficient yang floats atop. The lung, liver, heart, and spleen channels have all been invaded. The pathogenic factor comes from the kidneys. In this case, one must treat all the external and internal channels and collaterals by sedating feiyang (B58) on the foot taiyang channel and tonifying fuliu (K7) and dazhong (K4) on the foot shaoyin channel with acupuncture. In the jueyin excessive condition, the qi is deficient and there is pain and soreness in the heart. This excess qi, when lingering in the channels and collaterals, can induce sweats. In this case, one must regulate the diet to fortify and tonify along with the use of herbs. With acupuncture, one must needle taichong (LIV3) points on the jueyin channel."

Huang Di asked, "What does the taiyang pulse feel like?"

Qi Bo answered, "Taiyang represents the qi from the three yang. It is the major yang, and therefore the pulse floats. It is abundant."

Huang Di then asked, "What does the shaoyang pulse feel like?"

Qi Bo replied, "Shaoyang means lesser yang; thus it represents the formation of yang. This pulse is slippery but not strong."

Huang Di inquired, "What does the yangming pulse feel like?"

Qi Bo said, "The yangming pulse is big and floating. The taiyin pulse is deep, but under the fingers it pulsates with strength. The other two yin pulses are deep and not floating."

CHAPTER 22

SEASONAL ORGAN PATHOLOGY

Huang Di asked, "There is a concept of taking the principles that govern the five zang organs and applying them to the seasons and five elements in diagnosis and treatment. What determines the efficacy and failure of this?"

Qi Bo answered, "When we talk about the five elements, we are discussing the dynamics of the creative and control cycles, the changes of excess and deficiency, and so forth. By understanding the principles underlying these changes, we can apply them to disease progression. We can determine the severity of a problem and its changes on an hourly basis to the very time of death. We can analyze the success or failure of a treatment method."

Huang Di asked, "Would you please be more specific?"

Qi Bo patiently answered, "The liver corresponds to wood and to spring, and is coupled with the gallbladder. Therefore, spring is the most propitious time to treat problems of the foot jueyin/liver and foot shaoyang gallbladder channels. Liver and gallbladder correspond to the jia and yi of the energetic almanac in Taoist cosmology. These, too, are part of the wood element. On the jia and yi days of the sixty-day cycle in the almanac, the liver is at its highest point. The nature of the liver is to disdain constriction. Thus, one should consume sweet-tasting herbs to soften it.

"The heart corresponds to fire. It is dominant in the summer and is coupled with the small intestine. Summer is the best time to treat both hand shaoyin/heart and hand taiyang/small intestine. In cosmology they correspond to the bing and ding; the bing and ding days are the height of the heart. The heart disdains being scattered. One should consume sour herbs to keep the heart flow contained.

"The spleen corresponds to earth, is at its height in late summer, and is coupled with the stomach. Late summer is the best time to treat the foot taiyin/spleen and foot yangming/stomach channels. In cosmology they correspond to wu and ji, and they correspond to earth; these days are the height of earth within their sixty-day cycles. The spleen disdains dampness, so we must administer salty herbs to dry this damp.

"The lungs correspond to metal, connect to the fall, and are coupled with the large intestine. Autumn is the best time to address the hand taiyin/lung and hand yangming/large intestine channels. Gen and xin in cosmology are the days when lung energy is at its height, and these days are the most opportune times for treating the lungs. The lungs disdain upward, rebellious movement, so we must administer bitter herbs to purge and disperse.

"The kidneys correspond to water, come alive in the winter, and are coupled with the bladder. Winter is the best time to treat the foot shaoyin/kidney and foot taiyang/bladder channels. Ren and kui in cosmology are the days when kidney energy is at its highest. The kidneys disdain dryness, so we must use pungent and lubricating herbs. Pungent herbs will help to mobilize and dispense the body fluids to lubricate the body."

Qi Bo went on, "When the liver is diseased, it will naturally recover in the summer. If it does not, and disease progresses into the autumn, the condition will worsen. If the patient does not die in the autumn, the condition will not be curable in the winter. However, recovery is possible the following spring. In particular, one should avoid drafts. People with liver disease will typically recover by the bing ding days. If they do not recover on these days, they will worsen by gen xin days. If they do not die, then their condition will remain on ren quei days, until the return to the jia yi days of wood. Recovery will then occur. The spirits and minds of such patients are clearest at dawn. The condition will typically exacerbate toward evening, and then calm down by midnight. Those who suffer from liver illness respond to dispersing methods. One must therefore use pungent herbs. If they need tonification, however, the pungent tonics must be used for fortification. If they need sedation, sour herbs should be used.

"When the heart is diseased, it will recover in late summer. If this does not occur, it will worsen in the winter. If death does not occur, then the condition will remain the same in the spring, with recovery occurring the following summer. One should avoid eating hot foods and overdressing. Heart patients usually recover by wu ji day. If not, they will worsen by ren kui. If they do not die, they will suffer through the jia yi days. Finally, by the bing ding days, they may recover. Heart patients feel best by noon, but worsen around midnight. As day breaks the condition quiets down.

Heart disease should be cared for using softening methods. Salty herbs are utilized for this and for tonification. Sweet herbs are used to sedate.

"Disease of the spleen typically recovers in the autumn. If patients do not die in the spring, the disease remains into the summer. By the late summer, recovery occurs. One should avoid hot foods, overeating, and damp environments. Patients with spleen disease should recover by gen xin days. If not, disease exacerbates by jia yi days and remains through bing ding days. By wu ji days, recovery occurs. Spleen-diseased patients feel best in the afternoon and worst at daybreak. Conditions calm down in the evening. The spleen must be harmonized or tonified with sweet herbs but sedated with bitter herbs.

"With lung disease one should find resolution in the winter. If not, worsening occurs by the summer. If death does not occur, recovery will come in the autumn. One should avoid cold foods and underdressing. Lung patients should recover on ren quei day. If not, conditions will worsen on bing ding day. Disease worsens on wu ji days, with recovery finally occurring on gen xin days. Lung patients are most comfortable in early evening and worsen around noon. By midnight the condition quiets down. Lungs need to be converged or tonified with sour herbs; pungent herbs are used to sedate.

"Kidney disease can show recovery in the spring. If not, by the late summer it worsens. If death does not occur, conditions remain stable in the autumn, with recovery in the winter. One should avoid hot foods and drink, as well as clothes straight from fire drying. Kidney patients should recover by jia yi days. If not, they will worsen on wu ji days. If they are still alive on gen xin days, the condition remains stable. Finally, ren kui days bring remission. The most favorable time of day is the middle of the night. Aggravation occurs during chen, xu, chou, and wei hours (7–9 A.M. and 7–9 P.M., 1–3 A.M. and 1–3 P.M.). Calming down occurs in the early evening. The kidney requires solidifying. This is done with bitter herbs, which tonify as well. Salty herbs are used to sedate.

"When a pathogen enters the body, according to the principles and dynamics of the five elements, we can predict the rise and fall of both the antipathogenic qi and the pathogen itself. We can thus know how an illness will develop and how the body will respond. This allows us to issue a prognosis.

"With liver disease of an excess nature, one will find hypochrondriac pain radiating to the lower abdomen, and anger. When the disease is deficient, one will have blurry vision, some deafness, and fear, as if being hunted. In this case, acupuncture the jueyin and shaoyang channels. If liver qi rises to cause congestion in the head, headaches, deafness, and swelling in the cheeks, one should needle and bleed the jueyin or shaoyang channels.

"In excess heart conditions, one will find chest pain, rib pain, and fullness with pain radiating to the scapula and inner portion of the arms. When the condition is deficient, one will find chest and epigastric distension and fullness. Also, the trunk and low back will have pain with movement. Here one must acupuncture the shaoyin and taiyang channels. One should also bleed the jinjin and yuye points under the tongue. If the condition changes, needle and bleed the yinxi (H6) point.

"In excess conditions of the spleen, one will find heaviness, hunger, weakness of the muscles, difficulty walking, tightness in the tendons, and pain in the feet. Deficiency will manifest as abdominal distension, fullness, and borborygmus. There will be diarrhea with undigested food. One should needle and bleed points on the taiyin, yangming, and shaoyin channels.

"Excess conditions of the lung will manifest as asthma, shortness of breath, upper back pain, sweating, and pain or soreness of the lower extremities and genitals. In deficiency conditions shortness of breath, difficulty maintaining continuity of breathing, deafness, and dry throat will manifest. One should acupuncture the taiyin and foot taiyang channels. One should bleed the shaoyin channel.

"In excess kidney conditions, one will find swelling in the lower abdomen, asthma, dyspnea, sluggishness and heaviness, night sweats, and aversion to wind. In deficiency one will find chest pains, abdominal pain, clear urination, and unhappiness. One should acupuncture and bleed shaoyin and taiyin channel points.

"In general, dietetics is an extremely effective treatment for rectifying imbalance of the zang organs. Disease of the liver corresponds to a green complexion; one should eat sweet foods to soften the liver. This includes rice, beef, dates, sunflower greens, and greens.

"Disease of the heart corresponds to a red face, and sour foods should be eaten to contain the heart, including dog meat, plums, chives, and small beans like mung or adzuki beans.

"Disease of the lungs corresponds to a white complexion and one should eat bitter foods to help it disperse, such as wheat, lamb, apricot kernels, garlic, and onions.

"Disease of the spleen corresponds to a yellow and sallow face and one should eat salty foods to help dry dampness, such as black beans and soybeans, pork, chestnuts, and the leaves of a bean plant.

"Disease of the kidneys corresponds to a black and dark face. One should eat pungent foods to help it disperse, such as corn, chicken, peaches, and scallions.

"In general, foods that are pungent have dispersing qualities, those that are sour have astringent qualities, sweet foods have harmonizing and decelerating qualities, bitter foods have a dispensing and drying effect, and salty foods have a softening effect.

"When pathogens are strong, the physician should use medicinal herbs to attack and dispel. When the body is deficient, the physician should use dietetics to supplement and fortify. The five grains are used to nourish, the five fruits to assist, the five animals to fortify, the five vegetables to fulfill. Combining the energetic properties of these in one's diet can reinforce the essence and qi. These five types of food have specific effects and properties. When combined with the principles of the seasons, the five elements, and the pathophysiology of the five zang organs, one can utilize the methods of dietetics as an adjunct tool to nourish, convalesce, and treat."

CHAPTER 23

THE PARADIGM OF
THE FIVE ELEMENTAL PHASES

———

QI BO said, "The five flavors enter the stomach and are transported to the five corresponding zang organs. Sour corresponds to the liver, pungent to the lungs, bitter to the heart, sweet to the spleen, and salty to the kidneys. Each individual zang organ when diseased has its own symptomatology. The heart manifests in burping; the lung in coughing; the liver in talkativeness; the spleen in acid regurgitation; the kidney in yawning and sneezing; the stomach in vomiting; the large intestine and the small intestine in diarrhea and edema; the bladder in difficulty urinating or incontinence; the gallbladder in being easily angered. When the jing/essence qi of the five zang organs is overly concentrated in one area, instead of being stored in the individual zang organ, imbalance will occur. When the heart is overly abundant, symptoms such as hysteria or giggling will manifest; when the lung is overly abundant, grief and crying will manifest; when the liver is overly abundant it overacts on the spleen and there is an excess of worrying; when the spleen is overly abundant it overacts on the kidneys and there is a tendency toward being timid; when the kidney is overly abundant, there is a high degree of fright.

"Each of the five zang organs also has its aversion. The heart is averse to heat, the lungs to cold, the liver to wind, the spleen to damp, and the kidneys to dryness. They also have their corresponding body fluids. Sweat is the manifestation of the heart; mucus is the manifestation of the lung; tears are the manifestation of the liver; digestive fluid is the manifestation of the spleen; saliva is the manifestation of the kidneys.

"The five flavors have certain impacts on the body because of their natural properties; hence they have specific contraindications. Because pungent taste disperses qi, one should avoid eating pungent foods in diseases of the qi. Salty taste purges the blood. Thus in blood disease one should avoid salty foods. Bitter taste drains the bones, and thus should be avoided in bone diseases. Sweet taste bloats the flesh. Thus, in diseases of the flesh, avoid sweet foods. Sour taste contracts the tendons and should therefore be avoided in diseases of the tendons.

"There are also the five disorders and their times of occurrence. Yin illness generally manifests in the bones. Yang illness manifests in the blood. Yin illness generally manifests in the flesh. Yang illness generally manifests in the winter. Yin illness generally manifests in the summer.

"When the five zang organs are attacked by pathogens, there are the five pathologic manifestations within the body. For example, when the pathogen enters the yang level, one will become manic. When it enters the yin level, one will manifest bi or stagnation. When the pathogen is struggling at the yang level, one will manifest vertigo, dizziness, and problems of the head. When the struggle is at the yin level, one will become hoarse or lose one's voice. When the pathogen travels from the yang level to the yin, the symptoms will quiet down and the patient will become more withdrawn. When the illness travels from yin to yang, the patient will have outbursts of anger. These are the five pathologic disorders.

"There are also the five pathologic pulses. In the spring instead of the normally wiry pulse we see the floating pulse of the autumn. In the summer instead of the flooding pulse we see the sinking pulse of the winter. In the late summer instead of the slippery pulse, we see the wiry pulse of the spring. In the autumn instead of the floating pulse, we see the flooding pulse of summer. In the winter instead of the sinking pulse we see the slippery pulse of the late summer.

"The five zang organs have their corresponding attributes of spirit. The heart houses the shen, the governing spirit. The lungs house the po, or courage and boldness. The liver houses the hun, or intuition. The spleen houses the yi, or intellect. The kidney houses the zhi, or willpower and volition. They each dominate and control one area. The heart controls the blood vessels; the lungs, the skin and body hair; the liver, the tendons and nails; the spleen, the flesh and muscles; the kidneys, the bones and marrow.

"There are also the five overstrains one should avoid. Prolonged staring injures the blood; prolonged lying injures the qi; prolonged sitting injures the flesh and muscles; prolonged standing injures the bones; prolonged walking injures the tendons.

"The five zang organs should manifest pulses that correspond to the four seasons under normal circumstances. The liver pulse of spring should be wiry; the heart pulse of summer should be flooding; the spleen pulse of late summer should be slippery; the lung pulse of fall should be floating; the kidney pulse of winter should be sinking."

CHAPTER 24

—

CHANNEL CONSTITUENTS AND ACUPUNCTURE TECHNIQUES

—

Q I BO stated, "Within the human body, the amount of qi and blood varies from channel to channel. For example, the taiyang channel contains more blood and less qi. The shaoyang channel contains less blood and more qi. The yangming channel contains more qi and an abundance of blood. The shaoyin channel contains more qi and less blood. The jueyin channel contains more blood and less qi. The taiyin channel contains more qi and less blood.

"The foot taiyang/bladder and foot shaoyin/heart channels are externally and internally coupled channels. Other pairings are the foot shaoyang/gallbladder and foot jueyin/liver channels; the foot yangming/stomach and foot taiyin/spleen channels; these are the couplings of the three yin and yang channels of the foot. The yin/yang couplings of the hand are the hand taiyang/small intestine and hand shaoyin/heart; the hand shaoyang/sanjiao and hand jueyin/pericardium; the hand yangming/large intestine and hand taiyin/lung. We can trace illness in relation to the above couplings.

"Generally, when there is stagnation and fullness in the blood vessels, one should first utilize bloodletting to reduce symptoms and suffering. Next, observe the tendencies and relative strength of the patient before tonifying or sedating.

"In order to accurately locate the shu/transport points of the five zang organs on the back, the ancients used a strand of grass. The strand was the length of the distance between the nipples. This was folded in half, and another strand of this half-length was used to form an equilateral triangle. The top of the triangle was placed at dazhui (DU14), and the two lower corners then rested on the lung shu points. Moving the triangle down two vertebrae, one locates the heart shu points; four vertebrae further down will locate the liver shu; two vertebrae further down locates the spleen shu; and three vertebrae below this locates the kidney shu points.

"People who appear physically sound but who are depressed or bitter often develop conditions in the channels and collaterals. One should use acupuncture and moxibustion to treat this. People who appear physically and emotionally sound, but who tend to be overly joyous, develop problems of the flesh and muscles. One should also use acupuncture for this. People who seem joyous but appear physically unwell will often manifest conditions of the tendons and bones. One should use warming techniques of water bottles, baths and Dao-in. People who seem physically strained and emotionally depressed or bitter will manifest illness in the throat or have difficulty swallowing. One should use herbs for this. People who are repeatedly startled or traumatized have an obstruction of qi and blood in the channels and collaterals. They can manifest numbness or paralysis of the extremities. One should use tuina, massage, and herb wine in these cases.

"When acupuncturing the yangming channels one can apply bloodletting and sedation to disperse the excess qi. When acupuncturing the taiyang channels, one can let the blood out but should not allow the qi to escape. When acupuncturing the shaoyang channels, one can let the qi out but should protect the blood. When acupuncturing the taiyin channels, one should let the qi out but not the blood. When acupuncturing the shaoyin channels, one should also let the qi out but not the blood. When acupuncturing the jueyin, one should let the blood out but retain the qi."

CHAPTER 25

—

THE PRESERVATION OF HEALTH

—

H UANG DI asked, "Of all things under heaven, nothing is more precious than human beings. People are dependent on the nourishment and fortification of heaven and earth, water and food, and the essence of the universe to grow and prosper, according to the laws and changes of the seasons. This is true from royalty to the commoners. Every single person, without exception, has a desire to preserve his or her health. However, most people, throughout their lives, are plagued by disease in one form or another. Many times an illness begins when one is unaware of an imbalance that has subtly begun. This allows a pathogen to accumulate and degenerate the body, progressing to the point where it penetrates the level of the bones and marrow. Often at this level it is too late. It is my sincere desire to alleviate people's sufferings. Can you advise on how best to do so?"

Qi Bo replied, "Let me answer you with some examples. Salt stored in a container gradually seeps a fluid. This is the qi of the salt draining. A string on an instrument, on the verge of breaking, will display a brittle, high-pitched dying sound. A tree with shallow roots, although its branches and leaves are abundant, eventually will wither because its inside is empty. Certainly, when humans manifest conditions similar to these, we are told of severe damage to the internal organs. Because the skin, flesh, qi, and blood have become damaged and drained, it will be difficult to rejuvenate the person, even with the intervention of acupuncture, herbs, and moxibustion."

Huang Di said, "I have sympathy for the suffering of patients. But sometimes I hesitate and am unsure. After my treatments, patients occasionally get worse. However, I do not have a better way of treatment. Other people observing me may think I lack compassion. How do you advise me?"

Qi Bo answered, "Every individual's life is intimately connected with nature. How people accommodate and adapt to the seasons and the laws of nature will determine how well they draw from the origin or spring of their lives. When one understands the usefulness of the ten thousand things in the universe, one will be able to effectively utilize them for the preservation of health. The universe is comprised of yin and yang. The human being has the twelve channels. Nature exhibits hot and cold seasons; the human being has deficiency and excess. When one can manage the polarity changes of the universe, assimilate the knowledge of the twelve channels, and obey the rhythms of the four seasons, one will have clarity and not be confused by any disorder. Grasping the shifts of the eight winds and the transformation of the five elements, and understanding these in the context of a patient's health, you will gain insight into the truth. You could even disregard the obvious manifestations of the patient and attain, through the aforementioned, a transpiercing vision."

Huang Di asked, "The physical being of the human being cannot be discharged from the influence of yin and yang. In regard to various energy conditions of the universe, the ancient books have categorized on earth the nine continents and the four seasons. The moon waxes and wanes and days are long and short; in terms of the myriad things under heaven, it is impossible to completely measure and categorize the variations and changes. Within the human body, there are also many changes. What kind of method or framework can I use to understand and apply these principles of change?"

Qi Bo replied, "The principles of the five elements would help you understand all transformations in the universe. For example, metal can cut down wood; water can put out fire; wood can penetrate earth; fire can melt metal; earth can contain water. These transformations can be applied to the myriad things of the universe. In acupuncture one applies the same principles. In this way, one can bestow benevolence upon all people.

"There are five requisites for an effective practitioner. Most physicians ignore these five edicts. First, one must have unity of mind and spirit, with undistracted focus. Second, one must understand and practice the Tao of self-preservation and cultivation. Third, one must be familiar with the true properties and actions of each herb. Fourth, one must be proficient in the art of acupuncture. Fifth, one must know the art of diagnosis. When one follows these five edicts one will be effective. With acupuncture one can tonify the deficient and sedate the excess. But if one can observe the yin and yang laws of the universe and truly apply their essence to treatment, the results will be even better. This is like a shadow following a form. There is no secret here. It is that simple."

Huang Di asked, "Would you discuss the principles of acupuncture?"

Qi Bo answered, "The key to acupuncture is first of all to concentrate and focus. You must perceive the deficiencies and excesses of the organs, the variations of the three divisions of the body, and the nine pulses. Then you can administer acupuncture. You must also be able to detect whether the authentic zang pulse appears. This will allow you to determine if there are terminal tendencies of the zang, if the internal states match the external states. One cannot depend strictly on the appearance of the patient. One must emphasize the profound reading of the channels, blood, and qi in order to properly treat.

"Patients themselves can be categorized into excess and deficiency. When one encounters the five deficiencies, one must not be careless in the treatment. When one encounters the five excesses, one must not give up easily. In general, when it is time to withdraw the needles, pull them out quickly. Do not allow the time of a blinking eye to elapse. In therapy, one's every movement must be in concert; acupuncture should be smooth and even; the mind should be calm, the heart at ease. Observe the traveling of the qi with acupuncture to determine the best time to remove the needles. The arrival of qi, although not visible to the eye, is as if a flock of birds has converged. When the qi is leaving, it is as if all the birds in a flock have scattered simultaneously. You cannot find a trace of them. Thus, when acupuncturing, if the qi has not arrived, one should retain the needle as if one has drawn a bow in the ready position. As soon as the qi has arrived in the proper proportion, quickly remove the needle as if the arrow is being released."

Huang Di asked, "How do you treat deficiency and excess conditions?"

Qi Bo replied, "When treating deficient conditions, use the tonification method. When treating excess conditions, use the sedation method. The important thing is to make sure that the qi in the channels arrives. You must grasp the moment. Regardless of how deep or shallow the point, or whether it is distal or proximal, when acupuncturing you must focus your qi and your shen or spirit as if facing an abyss one thousand feet deep. Everything must be done with delicate care. When manipulating the needles with your fingertips, you should handle the needles as if handling a fierce tiger. Focus all your attention."

CHAPTER 26

—

ACUPUNCTURE IN ACCORDANCE WITH COSMIC CYCLES

—

H UANG DI said, "In acupuncture techniques, there are specific guidelines. Can you explain these guidelines and principles?"

Qi Bo answered, "In the context of the transformations of nature,
one must reflect and experience the art of healing."

Huang Di asked, "Please explain."

Qi Bo replied, "All methods of acupuncture must be in accordance
with the movements of the four seasons, the moon, the sun, and the stars.
These factors will impact the functions of the human body. During warm
weather and bright, cloudless days, blood flow is smooth. The wei/defen-
sive qi floats to the surface. Conversely, in cold, cloudy weather with little
exposure to the sun, the blood flow becomes choppy. The wei qi does not
flow to the surface as easily, and may sink within.

"During the new moon, the blood and qi also begin to flow more
easily. At the height of full moon, the blood and qi are full and the muscles
become strong. When the moon wanes, the channels and collaterals become empty of blood. Wei qi decreases during this time. The muscles
become less nourished. One must follow these changes of nature to properly regulate qi and blood.

"During the winter one should acupuncture less. When the weather
warms one can apply more acupuncture. During the new moon one should
not sedate. During the full moon one should not tonify. During the period
of no moon one should use less acupuncture. It is said that if one sedates
during the new moon, one will weaken the organs. If one tonifies during
full moon, one causes the blood and qi to overflow. This will cause stagnation of the collaterals. In the last quarter of the moon, acupuncture can
disrupt the qi flow in the channels. These are all examples of misapplication
and not observing cosmologic influences, which disrupt the balance within.
This misapplication facilitates the progression of illness to deeper levels."

Huang Di asked, "What is the significance of observing the positions of the constellations during various times of the seasons?"

Qi Bo replied, "One of the reasons to observe the constellations and stars is to determine the rise and fall and pathway of the sun and the moon. One can then predict and detect abnormal changes in the wind pattern. If a patient is already deficient, and is then invaded by the pathogens of the natural world, the condition will be compounded and the patient will suffer tremendous injury. Therefore, the physician who understands these principles can help prevent illness before it begins, prevent existing illness from worsening, or even allow some to rise from the dead. It is of utmost importance that one masters these principles."

Huang Di replied, "You are absolutely right. I now understand the prinicples of the constellations and seasons. I would like to know how we can emulate the ancient achieved ones."

Qi Bo said, "In order to tap the wisdom of the ancient achieved masters, one must read and understand the *Zhen Jing* [Classic of Acupuncture]. At the same time, one must master weather patterns, the waxing and waning of the moon, seasonal factors, and the tendencies of qi flow, to truly comprehend the wisdom of the ancients. The physican can benefit by applying this knowledge, coupled with observation and diagnosis of the patient. This careful study can yield keen vision and precognition of the development of medical conditions. One who is able to accomplish this will be of a higher level than the ordinary physician. One will have a transpiercing vision into the depths of the human body that are not externally perceptible.

"Xu xie, a weak pathogen, comes from nature. It is often a result of disharmony of weather patterns. Zheng xie, a strong pathogen, is the result of the patient being attacked while tired, weak, and with open pores. The strong pathogen tends to manifest mildly. Thus, most physicians do not detect it until it is severe. The highly developed physician, however, is able to detect illness in its infancy; he or she detects the tracks of the illness. In this case, the nine pulses of the three areas have not yet displayed changes. But still, the superior doctor begins the treatment. He or she knows how to carefully 'watch the door and the window in order to catch the thief.' The mediocre doctor, however, waits until the illness has taken hold to apply treatment."

Huang Di said, "I have heard of techniques of tonification and sedation in acupuncture. Can you please explain these to me?"

Qi Bo answered, "In employing sedation techniques one must grasp the concept of fullness. What is meant by fullness? This means that the patient's qi is full, that the moon is full, that the weather is full and warm. The patient must be calm and at ease; then acpuncture should be applied when the patient is inhaling. Wait until the patient inhales again to manipulate the needle; again, this is the idea of fullness. Wait for exhalation to withdraw the needle. In employing the sedation technique you must understand this concept of fullness, then utilize the technique to rid the body of the pathogen and restore the normal flow of zheng/antipathogenic qi.

"In employing tonification techniques one must grasp the state of roundness. What is meant by roundness? Round refers to flow, the flow of qi. This refers to guiding the qi to the place of deficit. One must puncture precisely and impact the ying, or nutritive, and blood. One must also wait for inhalation to withdraw the needle. A cultivated physician with mastery of techniques must understand the meaning of the patient's physical appearance and shape, size, and relative state of ying and wei, or nutritive and defensive, qi and blood in order to accomplish the intended purpose. The human body is so precious that one must pay the utmost attention with great care."

Huang Di exclaimed, "Wonderful! The way you have expounded on the transformations and changes of yin and yang, the seasons and cosmology, has enlightened me greatly.

"You have mentioned the physical appearance of the body and the shen. What exactly do you mean by body and spirit?"

Qi Bo answered, "I will talk about the body first. Observe, inspect, and diagnose the changes in the physical body. Feel through the pulses. What you cannot see, you ask about. In this way you will find the diseased or imbalanced parts of the body."

Huang Di asked, "What do you mean by shen, or spirit?"

Qi Bo replied, "Shen is something that you will recognize when you see it. The shen can be observed through the patient's eyes. But the true vision is through your own eyes. What you receive as messages, your heart will understand. You can then visualize the patient's condition in your mind. You can intuitively know what the problem is. You do not have to depend on language. This is similar to the nighttime, when no one sees anything; but you can see, as if the wind has blown away the fog and mist. This is the shen I refer to. You can confirm the shen by detecting the nine pulses of the three areas. But you do not have to depend on that. If you are developed, you can pierce beyond the physical and know the truth."

CHAPTER 27

PATHOGENS

HUANG DI said, "I've heard of the book called *Jiu Zhen* [The Nine Needles], which contains nine separate treatises. Yet you have taken these nine treatises and expounded upon them so that they are now nine times nine, or eighty-one chapters. I've finally grasped the essence, but still I have questions. The *Zhen Jing* [Classic of Acupuncture] discussed various methods of treatment, primarily locating the excess or deficiency of the body and then utiliziing left and right, up and down techniques to regulate; using the left to treat the right and the upper to treat the lower. I understand these concepts, which are based on internal disharmony between the ying/nutritive and the wei/defensive or qi and blood, but not the imbalances resulting from a pathogen entering the channels. I am interested in the treatment of illness due to pathogenic invasion of the channels and collaterals."

Qi Bo answered, "A well-rounded physician must have certain set principles in medicine and must also observe the changes in nature. For example, in heavens there are changes in the positions of the sun, the moon with its waxing and waning, and the constellations. On the earth there are the rivers, tributaries, and oceans. In human beings there are the channels and collaterals. These all influence each other. When the weather warms, the flow of the waters in the rivers becomes calm and easy. When the weather is cold, the flow of waters stagnates. When the weather is excessively hot, however, the waters in the rivers become abundant, and flooding results. If storms begin, further disasters occur. Similarly, an external pathogen invades the body. Cold causes the channel and collateral blood and qi to stagnate. Heat will cause the blood to flow very freely and rapidly. Excessive heat will cause the channels and collaterals to swell. This we can detect at the radial pulse. When we detect a large pulse, the pathogen is abundant and excessive. A small pulse means that the pathogen is passive and diminishing. If, at the radial pulse, one cannot detect whether the condition is of a yin or a yang nature, one should proceed to the next step, that is, to examine the nine pulses of the three positions. Once the problem is detected, one should immediately address it to prevent it from developing.

"When acupuncturing excess conditions, have the patient inhale as you insert the needle. Be careful not to cause the qi to reverse its flow, or rebel. Once the needle has been inserted, wait quietly but observingly for the qi to arrive. Leave the needle longer so the pathogen does not spread. When manipulating the needle to grasp the qi, also have the patient inhale. Ask the patient to exhale as you slowly withdraw the needle. At the end of the exhalation, the needle should be completely removed. In this way the pathogen will completely exit the body. This is called the sedation technique."

Huang Di asked, "How do we tonify deficient conditions?"

Qi Bo replied, "When acupuncturing to tonify, find the point and rub the skin there. Press down with your finger to disperse the qi in the channel. Massage the point to stir up its energy. Then ask the patient to focus attention. Press your finger upon the point and insert the needle. Wait until the qi flows to the point; when the qi flows freely in the channel, you may take out the needle. Use your right hand to withdraw the needle, closing the hole with your left hand so as not to lose the qi. As you insert the needle, have the patient exhale. At the end of the exhalation, the needle should be inserted. Wait for the qi very attentively. As soon as the qi arrives, have the patient inhale. Then remove the needle. This way the qi will not be lost. After the needle is removed, massage the area around the point. Thus, the zhen/true qi is retained within the body. This is called tonification."

Huang Di asked, "After diagnosing the presence of a pathogen, how does one proceed to eliminate it?"

Qi Bo answered, "When the pathogen travels from the luo collaterals into the main channels and lingers in the blood vessels, the battle is between the wei/defensive qi and the pathogen. The patient will feel fever or chills, and the qi within the vessels will rise and fall, depending on the circumstances of the battle. The pathogen will then begin to disperse and not linger in one particular place. When chasing the pathogen, the physician must first detect its location and then stop its progression. Acupuncture with sedation technique should be performed. However, do not confront the pathogen head on when it is strong. The reason for this is that when the pathogen is in full force, the body's zheng qi is weakened. To sedate forcefully at this time would further exhaust the qi of the channels. If you wait until the pathogen passes the location and then sedate, you will not achieve the purpose either. You would then cause the zheng/antipatho-genic qi to escape and leave the fort underguarded and thus invite defeat. Therefore, in order to stop the pathogen in its tracks, you must be patient and observant and wait for it to arrive. You insert the needle just before the pathogen arrives. This enables you to properly disperse. It is very intri-cate and delicate. If the needle is inserted too soon or too late, you will not reach the pathogen; you will also injure the body. Mastery of acupuncture is like using a bow and arrow: you must know the precise moment to unleash the arrow. Mediocre acupuncturists are like those who hammer a wooden nail, dull and imprecise. You must find the right moment, and without hesitation, but with clarity, then you insert the needle. This is how to hit the target and dispel the pathogen."

Huang Di asked, "Can you tell me more about tonification and seda-tion?"

Qi Bo answered, "When we talk about attacking the pathogen, this has to do with bleeding at the appropriate time. This allows us to drain the pathogen and help the wei qi to recover. As the pathogen enters the body, it does not have a specific direction of travel. If one pushes the pathogen, it will move forward. With correct knowledge, one can lead the pathogen to an area where its progression can be stopped. One can also confront and sedate it by bleeding."

Huang Di said, "I understand. What if the pathogen takes the body's zheng qi hostage, but the pulses do not change? How would you then detect its presence?"

Qi Bo replied, "You must carefully palpate the pulses in the three positions. Pay special attention to left and right, up and down. Observe several changes in strength and weakness. Then you will be able to detect the location of the pathogen and await its arrival, in order to attack. If you do not master the nine pulses of the three positions, you will not be able to differentiate the location of the illness: the upper, lower, or middle. You will not be able to determine whether the patient has any stomach qi remaining. Without understanding pulse diagnosis of the three positions, a doctor will not be able to effectively prevent disease. If the doctor sedates a deficient condition, this will cause chaos in the channels. One will not be able to restore the zheng/antipathogenic qi. If the doctor tonifies an excess condition, this will enhance the perversity of the pathogen and strip away the wei/defensive qi. This can turn a normally progressing condition into a dangerous condition. Tragedy and death can result. The doctor who does not understand this will not last long. Those who do not understand how to perfectly combine the attributes of nature and the human being, who injure the qi instead of eliminating the pathogen, are engaged in futility.

"When a pathogen invades the body, it does not initially have a direction. One can nudge it along, lure it to a place where it can be stopped, or attack and confront it. When these techniques are properly employed, the disease can be immediately remedied."

CHAPTER 28

THE NATURE OF EXCESS
AND DEFICIENCY

HUANG DI asked, "What is meant by excess and deficiency?"

Qi Bo answered, "Excess and deficiency describe the state of the pathogen and antipathogenic qi. When the pathogen is abundant, we call this an excess condition. When the antipathogenic Qi is insufficient, we call this a deficient condition."

Huang Di asked, "What are the further details of excess and deficiency?"

Qi Bo replied, "Let me give you an example using the lungs. The lungs dominate qi. Qi deficiency is due to a deficiency of the lungs. When the qi is rebellious, the upper body is excess and the lower body is deficient. There will be coldness of the feet. If the lung condition occurs during any season other than the season of its controlling element, fire, which is summer, the patient may live. If it occurs during summer, then there may be grave danger.

Huang Di asked, "What is meant by superexcess?"

Qi Bo answered, "Superexcess points to conditions of high fever and fullness and excess of the pulse."

Huang Di asked, "What method do you use to treat when the channels and collaterals are all in excess?"

Qi Bo answered, "Excess of the channels and collaterals means that the radial pulse is rapid at the cun position but slow at the chi position. One must target the luo collaterals and the channels in treatment. When a pulse is slippery, disease is progressing normally. If a pulse is choppy, the disease is progressing abnormally. When there is sufficient qi, the pulse becomes slippery or smooth; when death is imminent, the pulse is withering or choppy. By keeping each organ and the bones and flesh free-flowing, the abundance of jing and qi is ensured. One can then preserve one's health."

Huang Di said, "Can you explain the condition where the qi in the luo collaterals is insufficient, but where there is abundant qi in the main channels?"

Qi Bo replied, "In this case, at the cun position the pulse is slippery, but the skin above the chi level is cold. During the autumn and winter, this is considered abnormal, but during the spring and summer it is normal. When treating this, therefore, one must consider seasonal compatibilities and deficiencies of the illness."

Huang Di asked, "What about the opposite condition, when the channels are deficient and the collaterals are full?"

Qi Bo replied, "This points to the skin of the chi position feeling warm with a full pulse, whereas the pulse at the cun position is choppy. When this occurs in the summer or spring, it is not advantageous; in fact, the patient may die. When it occurs in the autumn or winter, it will heal."

Huang Di inquired, "How would you treat these two conditions?"

Qi Bo answered, "In the case of collateral fullness with channel deficiency, one should moxa the yin channels and acupuncture the yang. In the case of channel fullness with collateral deficiency, one should acupuncture the yin channels and moxa the yang."

Huang Di asked, "What is superdeficiency?"

Qi Bo answered, "Superdeficiency includes deficiency of channels, deficiency of qi, and deficiency at the chi position."

Huang Di asked, "How do you differentiate these?"

Qi Bo replied, "In qi deficiency, the patient speaks feebly. This is due to jing qi deficiency. Deficiency of the chi position means that the ying and blood are depleted. To sum up, in disease when the pulse remains slippery, it is a good sign. When the pulse turns choppy in disease, the indication is death."

Huang Di asked, "What is the prognosis of a condition where the cold factor suddenly rises upward, causing the channel to become excess?"

Qi Bo answered, "When you detect a pulse that is full and excess but also slippery, this indicates a favorable prognosis. When the pulse is excess but choppy, this is a bad sign."

Huang Di asked, "What does it mean when a patient has a strong, excess, and full pulse and cold hands and feet, but a feverish feeling in the head?"

Qi Bo answered, "If this happens in the spring or autumn, the patient will survive. If encountered in the winter or summer, the patient will die.

"There is another pulse, which is floating and choppy. If this is accompanied by fever, the indication is also death."

Huang Di said, "There is another type of patient who physically appears to be full and in excess. What is the meaning of this?"

Qi Bo replied, "This type of condition may demonstrate a cun pulse that is rapid and hard. But the skin of the chi position feels stagnant. There is a lack of correspondence. This problem can be either favorable or lethal. When favorable, the hands and feet are warm. When lethal, the hands and feet are cold."

Huang Di asked, "When a lactating mother with febrile disease manifests a pulse that is small, what is the prognosis?"

Qi Bo answered, "If the hands and feet are warm, the qi of the stomach is still present. The mother will live. If the hands and feet are cold, the stomach qi has been depleted and the prognosis is death."

Huang Di asked, "What is the prognosis for a lactating mother with wind heat, dyspnea, rapid breathing, the mouth open, and a very contracted shoulder? What kind of pulse would we expect?"

Qi Bo replied, "In this type of condition, the pulse would be full and large. If the pulse has a soft, gentle quality, however, the stomach qi is intact. If the pulse has a rapid and wiry characteristic, death is indicated."

Huang di asked, "What does it mean if one sees blood during dysentery?"

Qi Bo answered, "Dysentery with blood accompanied by fever is a poor sign; if accompanied by chills, it is a good sign."

Huang Di asked, "What is the meaning of dysentery with mucus?"

Qi Bo answered, "In this case, if the pulse is sinking, the patient will live. If the pulse is floating, the patient will die."

Huang Di asked, "What is the meaning of dysentery with both blood and mucus?"

Qi Bo replied, "When the pulse is uprooted and faint, the prognosis is poor. When the pulse is slippery and large, the prognosis is good."

Huang Di asked, "With dysentery, if there is no fever and the pulse is not uprooted, how does one arrive at a prognosis?"

Qi Bo answered, "Generally speaking, when the pulse is slippery and large, the patient has sufficient resistance. When the pulse is choppy and floating, the patient will die. The time of death is determined by the individual true zang pulses."

Huang Di asked, "Can you please tell me about the conditions of epilepsy?"

Qi Bo answered, "When the pulse is slippery and large, the illness will most likely be healed. If the pulse is hard, small, and rapid, the condition is incurable."

Huang Di asked, "What is the meaning of deficient and excessive pulses in epilepsy?"

Qi Bo replied, "When the pulse is deficient, the condition is treatable; when the pulse is excess, the condition is incurable."

Huang Di asked, "How do you differentiate the pulses and determine the prognosis in cases of diabetic exhaustion?"

Qi Bo answered, "If one detects excess pulses here, the illness may be prolonged, but it is curable. If the pulse is floating, small, and hard, then the longer the condition persists, the poorer the prognosis."

Huang Di said, "During the spring, when treating a patient with acupuncture, one should use the luo points of various channels. During summer, one should use the shu/stream points; during autumn, one should emphasize the he/sea points of the six fu; during winter, one should close off the body, using less acupuncture, while emphasizing herbs and food in treatment.

"This does not exclude the use of acupuncture and external techniques for various types of abscesses or tumors that may require immediate attention. In these conditions there may or may not be pain; sometimes you can locate it, sometimes you cannot. One should needle three times alongside the hand taiyin channel; one should also needle points along both sides of the neck. If you can locate the abscess or tumor in the armpit, and it is accompanied by fever, you must needle five times on the foot shaoyang channel. If after acupuncture the fever persists, one must acupuncture the hand jueyin/pericardium three times. The luo point, lieque (LU7), of the hand taiyin can be added three times, as well as the jianzhen (SI9) points three times. Acute abscess conditions with convulsion of the limbs, accompanied by severe pain and profuse sweating, are due to insufficient qi in the foot taiyang/bladder channel. Therefore, one should needle the pangguanshu (B28) points to the foot taiyang channel.

"When the abdomen suddenly distends and resists pressure, one should acupuncture luo points, zhizheng (SI7), of the hand taiyang channel, as well as the shenshu (B23) and alarm point of the stomach, zhongwan (REN12).

"In cholera one should needle along the lateral side of the shenshu (B23), zhishi (B52) point five times. Also use points weishu (B21) and wei-cang (B50).

"When treating anxiety, one should acupuncture points on the five channels. For example, needle the hand taiyin and hand taiyang five times; needle one time the zhizheng (SI7) point; needle jiexi (ST41) of the foot yangming/stomach once; needle zhubin (K9) of the foot shaoyin/gallbladder three times.

"When treating exhaustion syndromes, sudden syncope, hemiplegia, atrophy, or rapid respiration conditions that occur in obese patients, recognize that these are usually due to overindulgence in rich foods. If you encounter patients with chest and epigastric fullness and an obstruction condition, this is usually caused by emotional trauma. Separately, a case of sudden onset where the patient may pass out, lose hearing, or experience obstruction of bowel or urine is usually induced by chaos of the qi and blood within. Some of these syndromes, however, are not internally induced. Instead, they may be induced by invasion of exogenous wind; thus they may stagnate, linger, produce heat, and exhaust the flesh. Others manifesting chills, and including difficulty walking, may be caused by wind, cold, or dampness."

Huang Di said, "Jaundice, sudden pain, epilepsy, and hysteria are all due to rebellious qi moving upward, a state of disharmony amongst the five zang organs caused by obstruction of the six fu organs. Headaches, ringing in the ears, and obstruction of the nine orifices are usually caused by imbalances in the stomach and intestines."

CHAPTER 29

A DISCOURSE ON THE TAIYIN AND YANGMING CHANNELS

—

HUANG DI said, "The foot taiyin and foot yangming channels are coupled, as are the channels of the spleen and stomach. They represent the exterior and interior and have different imbalances and pathologies. What are the reasons for this?"

Qi Bo answered, "Taiyin is a yin channel, while yangming is a yang channel. Therefore, their circulation is of different placement and they go through different changes, mirroring the four seasons. Their imbalances can be induced by exterior or interior causes. The etiologies are different; hence the manifestations are also different."

Huang Di asked, "What are their differences?"

Qi Bo answered, "The yang represents the heavenly qi. It is responsible for the defense of the exterior. It is usually excess, abundant, and tough. Yin represents earthly qi. It is responsible for the nourishment of the interior. It is soft and tends to be deficient. When evil wind attacks, it will encounter the yang qi. When one loses balance in lifestyle and diet, it is the yin qi that is affected. When illness attacks from the exterior, it will travel through the yang portions of the body into the six fu organs. When illness manifests internally, it will travel in the yin portions of the body into the five zang organs. When the six fu are affected, one will see fever, restlessness, insomnia, and rapid dyspnea. When illness is in the five zang, one will suffer distension, fullness, obstruction of the bowel, and diarrhea. The pathophysiology is that the throat corresponds to heavenly qi, and regulating the breathing has to do with the exterior. The saliva corresponds to earthly qi, and swallowing has to do with the interior. The yang channels are vulnerable to wind. The yin channels are vulnerable to dampness. The qi of the three yin channels travels from the foot to the head and descends along the arms to the fingertips. The qi of the three yang channels begins

on the hands, travels to the head, and descends to the feet. Thus the pathogen that attacks the six yang channels will first travel up and then downward. The pathogen that attacks the six yin channels will descend first and
then rise. That is why when one is attacked by wind, the top portion is
affected first. When injured by dampness, however, the lower portion is
affected first."

Huang Di said, "When the spleen is disordered, one will lose the
normal function of the four extremities. Why is this?"

Qi Bo answered, "In order for the extremities to carry out their
proper functioning, nourishment from the stomach is required. But the jin
and ye or body fluids cannot reach the channels of the four extremities
from the stomach directly. They must go through the transformational
process provided by the spleen to be properly distributed. This is normal
physiology. When the spleen is disordered, it cannot effectively transform
and transport the jin ye/body fluids. The extremities then suffer a lack of
nourishment, which also includes the gu/food qi. Gradually, the muscles
and tendons atrophy and lose function."

Huang Di asked, "Why is it that the spleen does not correspond to an
individual season? Sometimes it is considered late summer."

Qi Bo replied, "The spleen's placement is in the middle. It is the
earth. In the divisions of the four seasons, the time of the spleen is the last
eighteen days of each season. It does not really have a distinct season of its
own.

"The function of the spleen is to transform and transport the essence
of food and fluids of the stomach. The symbology of the earth is to nourish
all things in nature. It is all-encompassing. It is responsible for nourishing
every single part of the body. This is why it does not correspond to any
one particular time. It has a hand in every element."

Huang Di asked, "There is a membrane that connects the spleen and
stomach. How is it that the spleen is able to transport the jin ye to the
stomach?"

Qi Bo answered, "The spleen channel of the foot taiyin is called major
yin and encompasses all three yin. The channel connects with the stomach
and spleen organs and circulates through the esophagus. This is why the
taiyin channel is able to take the jin and ye from the stomach and transport
them it to the three yin channels of the hand and food. The stomach channel of the foot yangming is the superficial couple of the spleen channel. It
is able to take the qi from the taiyin and transport it to the hand and foot

yang channels of the body. All the organs within the body depend on the spleen channel to transport acquired essence from the stomach. This is how the spleen channel of the foot taiyin carries out its function of transformation and transportation. When the extremities of the body are unable to receive the essence, they gradually degenerate and atrophy."

CHAPTER 30

—

DISORDERS OF THE
YANGMING CHANNEL

—

H UANG DI said, "A person suffering from disorders of the foot yangming channel will have an aversion to crowds of people and heat,
and will be easily startled by the sound of wood clapping, but will be
soothed by metallic sounds. Why is it that such a patient is averse to this
wood sound?"

Qi Bo answered, "Foot yangming is the channel of the stomach,
which corresponds to the earth. The aversion occurs because wood controls the earth."

Huang Di asked, "What about the aversion to heat and fire?"

Qi Bo replied, "Foot yangming traverses a great deal of the major
musculature of the body. Its channel contains an abundance of qi and
blood. When a pathogen invades from the exterior, it will cause febrile
disease. Therefore, an aversion to heat is created."

Huang Di inquired, "Why then the aversion to people?"

Qi Bo said, "When the qi in the foot yangming becomes stagnant and
unable to flow downward, a rapid dyspnea is induced, with fullness in the
chest. This type of fullness, restlessness, and discomfort will transform the
personality into a dislike of people."

Huang Di asked, "Some manifestations of this rapid breathing from
stagnation can cause death. But some patients do not die. Why is this?"

Qi Bo answered, "Stagnation of the qi in the channel, when it has to
do with the zang organs, will result in death. However, when it is limited
to the external channels, it will be symptomatic only and not terminal."

Huang Di said, "I have observed that in severe cases of yangming
disorder, a person can become delirious to the point of running about
naked, talking loudly, and not consuming food for several days. At the same
time, these patients are able to climb great heights and perform unusual
feats, things they cannot do under normal circumstances. Why is this?"

Qi Bo answered, "The four extremities contain an abundance of yang qi. When there is an excess of yang in the channels, great stamina results. Thus, the person is capable of physically overachieving."

Huang Di asked, "Why is it that they like to run around naked?"

Qi Bo answered, "It is not that they like to do so, but rather that they are feverish and very hot. They dislike covering themselves and aggravating the heat."

Huang Di inquired, "What about the behavior of cursing at people, singing, and talking loudly?"

Qi Bo replied, "When the yang pathogen is excess, it will attack the spirit and muddle the senses. Therefore, these people appear crazy and unreasonable, and lose their senses of norm and appetite."

CHAPTER 31

—

DISCUSSION OF FEBRILE DISEASE

—

Huang Di stated, "The types of febrile diseases we have discussed are considered to be shang han or cold-induced infectious illnesses. Some will be cured while others will be fatal. The time lapse between the onset of disease until death is usually six or seven days. The persons who heal do so in about ten days. What is the reason for this?"

Qi Bo answered, "The taiyang/bladder channel controls the surface of the body. Its channel connects with the du/governing channel at fengfu (DU16), the wind palace point. The du channel controls all the yang qi of the body. Therefore, taiyang is also considered a governor of the yang qi. When a person is attacked by the pathogens of wind cold, for example, the battle that occurs between the yang qi and the pathogen causes heat to manifest. This is similar to any kind of friction. Though the heat may be strong, if a person's antipathogenic qi is abundant and strong, it can easily dispel the pathogen. Thus, that person lives. However, if the person has yang deficiency, the wind cold pathogen can penetrate to the interior and damage the internal organs. In this case there is disorder of both internal and external. There is weak antipathogenic qi and a ferocious pathogenic factor, which together result in death."

Huang Di said, "I would like to hear more about the condition of shang han."

Qi Bo answered, "I will describe the clinical manifestations of shang han and their transference. On the first day of shang han the foot taiyang/ bladder channel is attacked. As taiyang controls the skin and body hair, this is the point of entry. The channel begins near the eyes and runs up the forehead, over the scalp, down the neck, and all the way down the back. Its luo channel connects with the kidneys. It continues down the thigh and leg to the little toe. This is why when wind cold invades the taiyang channel, stagnating the flow of qi, one will manifest headaches and stiffness and ache in the back. On the second day of shang han the pathogen is transferred to the foot yangming/stomach channel. This channel controls the musculature. Symptoms will occur along the channel, which begins near the eye and goes down the cheek, down the throat, chest, and abdomen, then down the thigh past the knee to the toes. In this case, symptoms may be seen along the meridian pathway such as dryness in the nose, pain in the eye, difficulty lying in any position, and fever. On the third day of shang han, the disease progresses to the foot shaoyang/gallbladder. The meridian begins near the eye and runs over the side of the head, down to the shoulders and hypochondriac area, where it connects with the luo channel of the liver. The symptoms will include earache, deafness, and pain in the ribs. What I have just described has to do with wind cold attacking the three yang channels. The disease here is still at relatively superficial levels. Thus, inducing sweating can resolve the problem.

"On the fourth day of shang han, the disease progresses to the foot taiyin/spleen channel, which begins at the medial big toe, runs up the medial leg and thigh, and continues upward over the lateral abdomen and rib area. Because the spleen is now involved, transformation and transportation are affected. This is why one will see distension and fullness of the abdomen, and difficulty swallowing. On the fifth day of shang han, the disease travels to the foot shaoyin/kidney channel, which runs from the sole of the foot over the ankle, up the medial leg, and finally runs upward over the center of the abdomen and chest to the clavicle. The pathogen has now exhausted the body fluids, and one manifests dry mouth and thirst. On the sixth day of shang han, the disease progresses to the foot jueyin/ liver. It traverses the channel from the lateral big toe, over the foot, up the medial leg and thigh, to the inguinal groove and ribs. The disease now impacts the liver's ability to mobilize the qi. This causes irritation and contraction of the scrotum. Hence, six days into the shang han disease, all three yang and all three yin channels have been invaded. The five zang and six fu organs have also become diseased. Tremendous deficiency of antipathogenic qi occurs, causing stagnation of the ying/nutritive qi and wei/defensive qi. These then fail to transport to nourish and defend the five zang organs. This is why, within six days, one may die.

"If the human body and the antipathogenic qi are strong and able to battle the pathogen, the illness will gradually be defeated. Generally, by about the seventh day, the patient will begin to recover. After another three to five days, the patient will completely heal.

"If the yang and yin channels are not simultaneously affected by wind cold, on the seventh day a taiyang disorder begins to heal. Headaches decrease. On the eighth day the yangming symptoms will cool off. By the ninth day shaoyang symptoms decrease and acute hearing is restored. On the tenth day the taiyin illness recedes. Distension and fullness return to normal, and appetite is restored. On the eleventh day shaoyin heals, wherein one can sneeze and not suffer from dryness and thirst. On the twelfth day the jueyin channel is able to disperse and relax again. The scrotum is no longer contracted and the lower abdomen is soothed. The pathogen has now been completely fended off."

Huang Di asked, "Will you please describe your treatment?"

Qi Bo said, "According to channel differentiation, when the patient has been affected for three days or less, one can induce sweating. This is because the pathogen is still at a relatively superficial level. After three days, when the pathogen has penetrated to the three yin channels, one should purge, in order to sedate and bring out the pathogen. These principles should, of course, be flexibly employed."

Huang Di said, "In some cases of febrile disease, although the illness is cured, there is some residual heat. Why is that?"

Qi Bo answered, "In general, patients have residual heat because during the severe part of febrile disease, they were force-fed food. The heat subsequently cannot be completely cleared. The pathogen must be cleared before much eating is done; otherwise food will be undigested and cause more heat."

Huang Di asked, "What is the method to clear this residual heat?"

Qi Bo answered, "Look at the patients' relative state of health, whether they are deficient or in excess. Give them proper treatment based on this to eliminate the heat completely."

Huang Di said, "What kind of food should one avoid during febrile disease?"

Qi Bo replied, "When such patients are fed animal products that are difficult to digest, a setback will occur. If they eat large quantities, too, this will cause more accumulation. Therefore, overeating or animal products should be avoided during febrile disease."

Huang Di said, "You mentioned a type of shang han which has affected both the yin and the yang aspects of the body, becoming terminal. Would you explain the mechanism behind this?"

Qi Bo answered, "In this illness, the patient contracts the wind cold pathogen in the yin and the yang channels simultaneously. On the first day the taiyang and shaoyin channels are affected. The patient has headache, thirst, irritability, and restlessness. On the second day the yangming and taiyin channels are affected. The patient feels abdominal distension, fever, lack of appetite, and delirium. On the third day the shaoyang and jueyin channels are affected. The patient experiences deafness, contraction of the scrotum, and coldness in the extremities. At this point, when the patient cannot consume liquids and is delirious, death will occur."

Huang Di said, "I have also seen that when the disease reaches a point where the five zang organs are impacted and the six fu organs are stagnant, the qi and blood do not flow. After three days, one will die."

Qi Bo replied, "The yangming channel is the most abundant with qi and blood. This is why when this channel is exhausted and drained, death can easily occur."

Qi Bo continued, "Febrile disease that begins with cold factors is termed wen bing when occurring before summer. When it occurs during or after summer, we call it shu bing. A summer pathogen should typically be dispelled with diaphoresis, and there should be no constriction of the sweating."

CHAPTER 32

—

ACUPUNCTURE IN THE
TREATMENT OF FEBRILE DISEASE

—

Qi Bo continued, "In febrile disease of the liver the patient will usually have symptoms of dark yellow urine, lower abdominal pain, fever, and hypersomnia. The patient may also suffer from headaches, dizziness, and vertigo, because the heat pathogen travels upward to the head through the liver channel, causing stagnation and obstruction of the head. At the moment of battle between the antipathogenic qi and the heat pathogen, we will see manic behavior and speech, distension, fullness or pain in the hypochondria area, restless limbs, and insomnia. On gen xin day the condition will certainly worsen. However, on jia yi day the patient will perspire and the fever will decrease. If the pathogen is strong and overcomes the organ, the condition will worsen and the patient will die on gen xin day. The treatment involves acupuncturing the foot jueyin/liver and foot shaoyin/kidney channels.

"Febrile disease of the heart will cause the patient discomfort and uneasiness for several days. Fever will then ensue. At the moment of battle the patient will have sudden chest pain, irritability, nausea and vomiting, redness of the face, and no sweating. The illness will get worse on ren kui day, and the fever will diminish, with perspiration, on bing ding day. If the pathogen overcomes the organ, the patient will die on ren kui day. Treatment involves acupuncturing the hand shaoyin/heart and hand taiyang/small intestine channels.

In febrile disease of the spleen there will be heaviness of the head, pain in the cheek area, restlessness, a bluish-green hue in the forehead, nausea, and fever. During acute flareup, or battle between good and evil, the patient might experience acute back pain and inability to bend the trunk of the body, distension and fullness of the lower abdomen, and diarrhea. On jia yi day the condition will worsen. If the pathogen overcomes the organ, the patient will die on that day. Otherwise, on wu ji day the patient will improve. Treatment involves acupuncturing the foot taiyin/spleen and foot yangming/stomach channels.

"In febrile disease of the lungs, the patient will have sudden chills and goosebumps, aversion to wind and cold, yellow coating on the tongue, and fever. During acute flareup one will have cough, asthma, dyspnea, pain radiating from the chest to the back, shortness of breath, severe headache, perspiration, and aversion to cold. On bing ding day the condition will worsen. If the organ is overcome by the pathogen, the patient will die on this day. If not, we can expect recovery on gen xin day. Treatment involves acupuncturing the hand taiyin/lung and hand yangming/large intestine channels. Let out a drop of blood the size of a pea. This should help recovery.

"In febrile disease of the kidneys one will see back pain, soreness of the calves, thirst, a desire to drink, and fever. During acute flareup the neck becomes stiff and painful, there is coldness in the calves, fever and flush in the soles of the feet, and a dislike of speaking. In the kidney qi rebels upward, one will have severe neck pain and vertigo. On wu ji day exacerbation will occur. If the pathogen overcomes the organ, the patient will then die. If not, recovery will occur on ren kui day. Treatment will involve acupuncturing the foot shaoyin/kidney and foot taiyang/bladder channels.

"In all the above-mentioned cases, those days when perspiration occurs and fever diminishes are those when energy is circulating most abundantly in the corresponding organ. This is like adding fresh troops to an ailing army. The pathogen can then be overcome and the patient will recover.

"In febrile disease of the liver, one will notice a red color on the left cheek first. In febrile disease of the heart, one will notice redness of the lips. In febrile disease of the spleen, one will see redness of the nose. In febrile disease of the lungs, one will see redness of the right cheek. In febrile disease of the kidneys, one will see redness just below the cheeks. In these instances, the color will appear before the disease manifests. Acupuncture can be administered to the patient immediately; this is called treating disease before it occurs.

"If illness has just begun, we will see it manifesting in the corresponding zang organ locations. If the pathogenic invasion is shallow and we do not see any other symptoms, treatment can be administered. By the most optimal day of organ correspondence, recovery will occur. If the wrong treatment is rendered, tonification instead of sedation or vice versa, the illness will be prolonged. You will then have to wait beyond three weeks for recovery. If you make a mistake again, you will have planted the seed of death. In general, in febrile disease one should induce sweating. Grasp the correct principles and wait until the right day and the right moment. The patient will then rain sweat and you will be victorious.

"When treating febrile disease, provide cooling drinks to cool the interior first, then administer acupuncture. Keep the environment cool and do not overdress the patient. This will eliminate the heat on the outside as well. If febrile disease begins with pain in the chest or hypochondriac area, or restless limbs, this is because the condition has its origin in the shaoyang channel. Acupuncture the shaoyang channel to dispel or sedate the heat in the yang portion. Tonify the foot taiyin channel as well, to check the pathogen. If the problem is severe, employ the 59-point method.*

"The above points can help to disperse or drain from the body any heat pathogen that is traveling upward.

"When febrile disease begins and one suffers from pain in the arms, the illness is in the upper body and has its origin in yang. Treat by acupuncturing the hand yangming/large intestine and hand taiyin/lung channels. Induce sweating to reduce the fever.

"Febrile disease that begins in the head is considered to be taiyang in nature. Therefore, acupuncture this channel for relief. A febrile condition that begins in the thigh has its origin in the lower body and is yang. Needle the foot yangming/stomach channel for relief. Febrile disease that begins as heaviness of the body, joint pain, deafness, fatigue, or hypersomnia has its origin in the yin. Needle the foot shaoyin channel. If it is severe, utilize the 59-point method. When febrile disease begins with dizziness, vertigo, fever, and chest and hypochondriac fullness, the origin is in the shaoyang/gallbladder channel. This is a half-interior, half-exterior condition, which will next travel internally. Acupuncture foot shaoyin/kidney and foot shaoyang/gallbladder points to direct the pathogen back out.

"Febrile disease of the taiyang/bladder channel displays flushing of the cheeks. If the redness is not too deep, the illness is mild and shallow. With proper treatment the pathogen will be dispelled on the day when sweating occurs. If the shaoyin/kidney channel is also infected, the patient will die in three days. Here the pathogenic heat has injured the kidneys. In shaoyin

*The 59-point method for febrile disease is discussed in depth in chapter 61.

channel conditions alone, the redness will manifest below the cheeks. In mild cases recovery will occur on the day when sweating occurs. If the jueyin channel is also infected, injury is caused to the liver and the patient will die within three days.

"When treating febrile disease, there are some important points. The point below the third thoracic vertebra is used to treat heat in the chest. The point below the fourth thoracic vertebra is used to treat diaphragm heat; the point below the fifth treats liver heat; the point below the sixth treats spleen heat; and the point below the seventh thoracic vertebra treats kidney heat.

"In treating febrile disease, one should acupuncture points in the upper portion of the body in order to rid the yang pathogen. Use points in the lower portion to tonify the yin. In the lower portion, use points near the tailbone, such as changqiang (DU1). Observe the facial colors in order to detect illness of the abdominal viscera. If the redness of the cheeks travels from the lower to the upper portion, the condition is called da jia xie, a type of dysentery. If the redness moves downward on the cheek, this indicates abdominal distension and fullness. If we see the redness behind the cheekbone, rib pain is indicated. Any color we observe above the cheek indicates illness above the diaphragm."

CHAPTER 33

—

A DISCOURSE ON WEN BING

—

HUANG DI said, "In wen bing or febrile disease, after the induction of sweating the fever should decrease, the pulse should quiet down, and the body should cool. But in some cases, immediately after the patient perspires the fever rises again, the pulse continues to be rapid, and the patient is delirious and cannot consume food. What is this condition called?"

Qi Bo answered, "This is called yin yang jiao. This means the yang pathogen has entered the yin level and become intertwined. This is considered terminal."

Huang Di inquired, "Why is this?"

Qi Bo answered, "The mechanism underlying this begins with perspiration. Sweat comes from the food and liquid that are consumed. Food and liquid depend on the jing/channel qi of the zang fu organs to transform and transport. In the battle with a pathogen, the pathogenic qi leaves with the sweat. In this case, the spleen and stomach are restored to normal functioning, the appetite returns, and the fever will not come back. However, if the fever does return, it means that the pathogenic qi was not completely eliminated. We can say that the antipathogenic qi is defeated and weakened. In order to support the antipathogenic qi, one must consume food and liquid. Without an appetite, this function is depleted—the more sweating, the more depletion. With the antipathogenic qi depleted and the pathogen growing in strength, the prognosis is death. If one perspires but the pulse remains excess and irritable, death is also indicated. This indicates that the antipathogenic qi is in defeat and on the verge of collapse. Delirium indicates that the spirit is disrupted and not housed by the heart. This is grave. The inability to eat indicates the exhaustion of stomach qi. This implies graveness, too. All three aspects point to a bad prognosis. Even if the condition appears to be improving, this is an illusion."

Huang Di said, "When people are sick with fever, they often feel irritable and full. This irritability is not relieved by sweating. What kind of illness is this?"

Qi Bo replied, "Fever and perspiration are symptoms of a taiyang condition. The irritability after perspiration is due to cold rising from the shaoyin channel. This condition is called feng jue, obstruction induced by wind."

Huang Di asked, "Can you please provide me with a more detailed explanation of this?"

Qi Bo answered, "Taiyang governs the surface qi of the entire body. When a pathogen invades, therefore, it will attack the taiyang first. Foot shaoyin and foot taiyang are coupled meridians. When taiyang is attacked by wind, leading to fever and sweating, this indicates the exterior is deficient. In this case, the cold energy from shaoyin will rebel upward and fill the taiyang meridian, causing stagnation and fullness of the chest."

Huang Di asked, "How do you treat this?"

Qi Bo answered, "Needle the taiyang and shaoyin points. Combine this acupuncture with herbal medicine."

Huang Di inquired, "Can you tell me about the syndrome of lao feng?"

Qi Bo replied, "Lao feng means attack of wind under physical duress. It occurs in the lower portion of the lungs. The patient suffers from a cough so severe it appears as if the eyeballs will pop out; also, blurry vision, chest fullness and pain, a thick, tenacious mucus, difficulty lying in a supine position, insomnia, chills, aversion to wind, and fever. The mechanism here is exhaustion, depletion, and duress, rendering the antipathogenic qi vulnerable. This allows wind heat to attack, stagnate, and congest in the lower part of the lungs."

Huang Di asked, "How is this condition treated?"

Qi Bo answered, "First, one must relieve the difficulty breathing. To do so, one must lure the wind heat out of the taiyang. The prognosis is that young people can recover in three days, middle-aged people in five days, and older people in seven days. The body's antipathogenic qi decreases with age. If the phlegm and pus are not expectorated, they will remain in the lungs and rot the lobes."

Huang Di said, "People with shen feng, or kidney wind, suffer from facial edema and a tongue so swollen that speech is affected. Can this condition be treated with acupuncture?"

Qi Bo answered, "If they are very deficient, acupuncture is contrain-

dicated. It may deplete the qi even more. A patient inappropriately acu-
punctured will be attacked by pathogenic qi within five days."

Huang Di asked, "What will they then feel?"

Qi Bo replied, "They will experience shortness of breath, fever, heat
radiating from the chest and upper back to the head, sweating, a feverish
feeling in the palms, dry mouth, great thirst, concentrated yellow urine,
swollen eyes, borborygmus, heaviness and swelling of the whole body, poor
mobility, irritability, no appetite, an inability to lie in a supine position,
cough, or amenorrhea in women. This condition is called feng shui."

Huang Di asked, "Would you please explain this?"

Qi Bo answered, "Because the antipathogenic qi is weak, the pathogen can attack the body. When there is yin deficiency, a yang pathogen
will invade. When heat first attacks the skin, it causes fever, sweating, and
shortness of breath. Yellow urine is due to heat attacking the taiyang channel. Not being able to lie prone is due to water retention affecting the
stomach. This pushes against the lungs and causes coughing. Water retention occurs first in the upper portion of the body, particularly the eyes."

Huang Di asked, "Why?"

Qi Bo replied, "Water is a yin factor. The eyes are considered yin, as
is the abdomen. Thus, the eye sockets and abdomen are simultaneously
affected by this swelling. The kidneys, impacted by the water pathogen,
cannot disperse their yin up to balance the heart fire. The heart fire, obstructed by the water, cannot move downward to balance the kidney water.
One will therefore manifest dryness, a bitter taste in the mouth, and thirst.
As the water pathogen moves upward it affects the lungs, causing coughing
with profuse, clear, watery phlegm. This is exacerbated by lying in a prone
position. The water also remains in the intestines, creating gas and borborygmus. The water also invades the spleen, impairing transformation and
transportation. One is then irritable and cannot eat. Because the stomach is
filled with water, one cannot take in food. The stomach meridian runs
down the leg. The water coursing down the channel causes one to feel
heavy or immobilized. The heart meridian connects to the uterus and re-
lates to menstrual function. As the water pathogen obstructs the heart and
lungs, their energy cannot move downward. Thus, the heart blood cannot
move properly to the uterus. Circulation of blood, qi, and water becomes
a problem, and amenorrhea results."

CHAPTER 34

———

IMBALANCES

———

HUANG DI said, "In certain instances, febrile diseases are not induced by exposure to heat pathogens from the exterior. However, febrile disease still develops. Why is this?"

Qi Bo answered, "This is because the yin of the body is deficient and the yang becomes relatively excess, thus causing an imbalance that manifests as fever and restlessness."

Huang Di said, "In certain instances, chills and cold occur not because of exposure to external cold or lack of clothing and protection. It is also not because coldness exists naturally within the body. Rather, this coldness seems to be produced by the body. What is the cause of this?"

Qi Bo replied, "Patients such as these primarily have bi conditions and tend toward stagnation, with a deficiency of yang. The yin becomes relatively excess and causes cold."

Huang Di said, "There is a condition where one has fever in the extremities only. When one is exposed to wind cold, the fever becomes exacerbated to the extent that one feels as if on fire. What is the reason for this?"

Qi Bo answered, "This type of patient is lacking in yin, with an excess of yang. Extremities are considered yang. When they are exposed to wind, the yin qi is depleted and the yang increases relatively. The lack of yin cannot balance the yang. Because of this excess yang, growth is diminished and atrophy develops."

Huang Di asked, "I have seen patients who experience chills although they bathe in hot water or sit by a fireplace. Even with added clothing they remain cold, although they do not shiver. What condition is this?"

Qi Bo replied, "In this type of patient the kidney qi tends to be susceptible to stimulation. The patient generally spends much time in water or works in a damp environment or indulges in excessive sexual activity as well as too much alcohol and caffeine. These deplete the kidney water/

yin, which in turn results in uncontrolled fire to dry out the marrow and jing/essence. Because the bones are hollow from lack of marrow, the coldness is felt to the bone level but because of the fire, one is cold in the bones but does not shiver. This condition is called gu bi, or stagnation in the bones, and it creates deformity and joint immobility."

Huang Di said, "Some people suffer from numbness. What kind of illness is this and why can't they feel?"

Qi Bo answered, "This is because there is a deficiency of the ying and wei, or the nutritive and defensive. The ying qi and blood are depleted and unable to nourish the skin and flesh. The wei qi is deficient and cannot warm and mobilize the extremities. This combination results in numbness or paralysis, although visually the extremities show minimal change."

Huang Di inquired, "I have heard that some patients are fine when standing or sitting, but wheeze in a prone position. Others breathe coarsely upon exertion and still others have difficulty sleeping. Can you tell me what organs are involved in these cases?"

Qi Bo answered, "In the case of one who cannot sleep and also wheezes at night, the yangming or the stomach qi is rebelling upward. Normally the qi of the three yang channels of the foot flows downward.

"The stomach is a receptor of foods and fluids. Stomach qi should move down to benefit the other organs. The stomach's function is to transport, not store. When the stomach qi rebels upward, the transformed products of the stomach stagnate. Over time, they turn into phlegm. The phlegm courses upward with the stomach qi, congesting the lung and heart. Thus, the patient cannot lie flat, and wheezes. If the phlegm disturbs only the heart and not the lung, there is trouble sleeping but there is no wheezing. As the ancient classic *Xia Jing* (Classic of Medicine) stated, when the stomach is in disharmony, one cannot sleep peacefully at night.

"If one has a normal daily life but wheezes, this is because the qi in the luo channel of the lung is rebelling upward. The luo channels are small and traverse the body as connectors, rather than flowing as large channels. This is why normal activity and sleep are not affected.

"When one cannot lie flat without experiencing asthma, it is due to water stagnation. Water is normally processed as jin ye and circulated throughout the body before excretion via the kidneys. When the kidneys are diseased and the bladder cannot excrete, water stagnates. Then it moves back upward and distresses the lungs and bronchioles. When the patient lies down, the water blocks off the bronchioles, causing asthma. Kidney yang is deficient and cannot transport the water. Yang is depleted through movement, and this is why dyspnea results from exertion. The lung dominates respiration, while the kidney grasps the qi. In kidney yang deficiency the qi is not grasped and rebels upward, resulting in asthma.

"In the case of one who has wheezes whether sleeping or moving, the kidneys cannot grasp qi and have water stagnation. In conclusion, for both the patient who cannot lie in a prone position without asthma, and the patient who cannot move about without asthma, the kidneys are much involved."

CHAPTER 35

—

MALARIA-LIKE ILLNESSES

—

H UANG DI stated, "In general, all malaria-like illnesses are caused by wind pathogens. The illnesses themselves, however, are very distinct as to flareup and remission time factors. Why is this?"

Qi Bo answered, "When one is having an attack of malaria, first one will get goosebumps, the hair will stand on end, and there will be discomfort of the extremities, a desire to stretch out, uncontrollable yawning, chills and shaking, tremors in the lower jaw, and back pain. Then the attack of chills will pass, followed by fever, splitting headache, and thirst, with a desire to drink cold liquids."

Huang Di asked, "What kind of pathogen causes such vicious manifestations?"

Qi Bo replied, "This is due to the pathogen and the body battling from bottom and top. There is also a great fluctuation between deficiency and excess. And as the body's yang is overcome by the pathogen, it creates an imbalance of excessive yin. When the yang qi is deficient in the yangming channel, there will be chills and shaking, even to the point where the lower jaw trembles. When the yang qi of the taiyang channel is deficient, there will be back pain and headache. If all three yang channels are deficient, the yin will dominate. When the yin dominates, there is coldness and pain within the bones and marrow. However, when the yin is overcome by the pathogen, it creates a condition of yang excess; hence, when the yang is excess, one will have fever. The heat is so extreme that one experiences dyspnea, thirst, and a desire for cold liquids to cool the insides. This is in part caused by summer heat, where the heat pathogen is dormant and hides just beneath the skin. It surrounds the intestines and stomach, where the ying or nutrients travel. Inside, one is like an enclosed swamp, stale and stagnant. As soon as the coolness of autumn arrives one is exposed and suddenly attacked by wind, particularly after bathing when the pores are open. The wind and moisture enter and harbor just beneath the skin where the wei/defensive qi travels. During the day wei qi travels at the yang level; during the night it travels at the yin level. If the pathogen is of yang nature it will likely manifest on the exterior; if the pathogen is of yin nature it will manifest within. The yin and yang battle between the inside and outside, causing an episodic attack of symptoms that represents the disharmony between both yin and yang."

Huang Di asked, "Sometimes malaria will flare up, then settle down for a few days before flaring up again. Why is this?"

Qi Bo answered, "The pathogen has lodged in a deeper part of the body, the yin part. This causes the yang qi and the yin qi to battle so deeply within that they do not manifest on the outside. The patient therefore experiences an attack every other day, because the pathogen is deep, close to the five zang organs. It is separated by the membranes of the abdominal cavity. Here it is farther from the wei qi, which therefore cannot engage the pathogen. It is only every other day that the wei qi can actually do battle with the pathogen."

Huang Di said, "Some malaria-like conditions will manifest the acute phase a little later with each succeeding day. Why is this?"

Qi Bo answered, "When the pathogen enters at the fengfu point (DU16), it moves down the spine through the vertebrae, one at a time. The wei qi, however, circulates once each day, finally converging at fengfu (DU16). Because the pathogen is traveling methodically downward, its attack manifests slightly later each day. After twenty-five days the pathogen reaches the coccyx. On the twenty-sixth day the pathogen penetrates deep into the spine. It then enters the chong/vitality channel. It follows the chong channel upward for nine days; it then emerges at quepen (ST12). From the point of entering the chong channel, and the upward movement, the episodic attacks reverse and begin to occur earlier each day."

Huang Di said, "You mentioned that whenever the wei qi circulates through fengfu (DU16), the palace of wind, the gate opens up and the pathogen can then enter, giving rise to the attacks of symptoms. Now you say that the wei qi and pathogenic qi do battle at points below fengfu (DU16) on the spine each day, thus giving rise to the attack of symptoms. I do not understand why there is a difference in location of battle between wei qi and the pathogen."

Qi Bo replied, "This has to do with the pathogen entering the body through the head and neck area and following the spine down. Each person has different resistance, even at different points of the body. The pathogen does not enter every person at fengfu (DU16). When the pathogen enters the body through the head and neck, and the wei qi engages it there, an acute attack occurs. If the pathogen enters through the upper back, however, the acute attack does not occur until the wei qi circulates to that area. This is true whether the pathogen enters through the lower back or the hands and feet. When the wei qi engages the pathogen at its point of entry, an acute attack occurs. Wind pathogens, of course, have no predictable area of entry. Wind catches the moment when the pores are open, and it is the point where the wei qi converges with the pathogen that the battle takes place and the disease manifests."

Huang Di said, "Malaria and wind disease seem very similar. Why is it that wind conditions persist continually, but malarial conditions have intermittent breaks?"

Qi Bo answered, "The wind pathogen lingers at the entry location, so one always has symptoms. The malaria pathogen, however, flows with the channels and collaterals. Only when it engages with the wei qi does an acute attack come about."

Huang Di said, "Some conditions of malaria, in its acute attack, will manifest chills and then fever. Why is this?"

Qi Bo answered, "During summer one may contract severe summer heat and suffer profuse sweating. If one is exposed to cold and damp at the time of sweating, these lodge in the body under the skin. By the arrival of autumn, one is vulnerable to the wind pathogen. This initiates the process of malaria. We can say that cold and water are yin pathogens; wind is a yang pathogen. The cold and water generate chills, the wind generates fever. We call this cold malaria."

Huang Di asked, "Can you discuss the type of malaria where fever precedes the chills?"

Qi Bo replied, "Here one is attacked by wind first. Exposure to water and cold follows. This is called heat malaria."

Huang Di said, "Will you please tell me about the type of malaria where there is fever but no chills?"

Qi Bo answered, "This occurs when a patient has a preexisting yin deficiency. Because this results in a yang predominance, the malaria attack manifests with shortness of breath, fullness, restlessness, feverishness of the extremities, and nausea. We call this dan malaria, an extreme heat type of malaria."

Huang Di said, "The ancient medical classics state that in excess conditions one should sedate, while in deficient conditions one should fortify. Here we are faced with fever, an excess manifestation, and chills, which indicate deficiency. The chills of malaria are such that bathing in hot water or sitting by the fire do not warm the patient. The fever of malaria is such that even bathing in ice water does not cool one down. These seem like excess and deficiency. Even very good doctors cannot successfully treat this at the time of acute attack. They wait for the period of remission before employing acupuncture. Can you elaborate on this?"

Qi Bo answered, "In the ancient medical classics, it is advised that during very high fever one should not utilize acupuncture. This is true when the pulse is chaotic or sweating is profuse. This is because when the pathogen is at its height, the body's energies flow in reverse. This is similar to the art of war; when the enemy is thoroughly prepared and in highest energy, one should not initiate battle. One should wait instead for the inevitable decline before proceeding.

"In the beginning of an acute malaria attack, the yang enters the yin level. The yang is now deficient and the yin is excess. Because the yang is deficient on the surface, there are chills and shaking. At the extreme manifestation of yin, the yang will emerge. When yang does this, the yin is deficient, the yang having become excess. Fever and thirst now appear. Either yin or yang will dominate and exhaust itself, allowing the other to take over.

"Malaria has to do with pathogenic wind and cold. Yin and yang manifest themselves to the extreme. They continually start and stop. With each recurrence the severity is like a sudden storm. This is why the ancient medical classic states, 'When the pathogen is at its peak, do not attack. If one attempts to attack, the patient's antipathogenic qi will become injured. Wait until the pathogen is waning. This is the method for success.' It is this reasoning that applies to treatment of malaria."

Huang Di said, "Excellent indeed. Can you please tell me, then, how does one treat malaria? And how does one grasp the principle of treating according to different times of the day?"

Qi Bo replied, "When malaria begins to flare up, it will start at the extremities. If the yang energy has already been injured, the yin will be affected as well. Before the flareup, therefore, one should tie the ten fingers with string. This way, the pathogen cannot enter more deeply and the yin energy cannot come out. After tying the fingers, observe the luo channels. Where purple stagnation appears in the capillaries, perform bloodletting.

This is called 'ambushing the enemy before being confronted.' This is before the body's qi engages the pathogen."

Huang Di asked, "When malaria is not in acute flareup, what conditions do we see?"

Qi Bo replied, "The pathogen within the body will eventually cause the yin and yang to be depleted. If the pathogen is at the yang level, one will have fever and a rapid, full pulse. If it is at the yin level, one will have chills and a quiet pulse. If both yin and yang are exhausted, the wei qi and pathogenic qi separate. The condition then arrests; but when wei qi engages the pathogen again, flareups recur."

Huang Di asked, "Can you tell me about the malaria condition that flares up every two days or on some regular basis? In this instance, some experience thirst while others do not. What is the reason for this?"

Qi Bo answered, "This type of skipping days between flareups occurs because the pathogen and wei qi usually engage at fengfu (DU16); sometimes they meet, however, only every two days. This causes the attack. Thirst is dependent on the severity of the disease and whether yin or yang dominates."

Huang Di asked, "In the ancient medical classics it is stated that in the summer one is injured by summer heat; then in the autumn one will experience malaria. Some malaria conditions, however, are not caused by this pattern. Can you please explain this to me?"

Qi Bo answered, "Some malaria conditions are different; they are contingent upon a seasonal perversity. For example, if the acute flareup is in the autumn, there are more chills. If the flareup is in the winter, the chills are not severe. If the flareup occurs in the spring, there is a strong aversion to wind. If the flareup occurs in the summer, there is profuse sweating."

Huang Di asked, "Can you please explain the wind or heat malaria and the cold malaria? How does the pathogen enter the body and what organs are affected?"

Qi Bo replied, "The heat type occurs like this: in the winter one contracts wind cold, which lodges in the marrow. In the spring, yang qi becomes active, but the pathogen does not travel outward until summer, when heat exhausts and stirs up the marrow. Muscles emaciate from the pores opening. If one then overstrains, the pathogen manifests itself as sweating. This pathogen lies dormant in the kidneys. During a flareup it rises up and outward with the sweat. This type of condition occurs because the yin is deficient and the yang is excess. Fever is the result. At its extreme point the pathogen reenters the yin level and chills result. Thus, fever and chills characterize heat malaria."

Huang Di asked, "Can you tell me about the extreme heat type of malaria?"

Qi Bo replied, "This is due to the fact that the lungs have a predisposition to accumulating excess heat. This heat becomes stagnant. Overstrain then opens the pores and wind cold attacks beneath the skin. This causes the condition to flare up. Here the yang is excess, so one sees fever but not chills. There are no chills because the pathogen has not entered the yin level. In this condition the pathogen can lie dormant in the heart. When it manifests, it travels in the muscles and flesh. If it lingers, the muscles emaciate. This is the mechanism of dan ji, or heat malaria."

CHAPTER 36

—

ACUPUNCTURE IN THE
TREATMENT OF MALARIA

—

Qi Bo stated, "Malaria conditions that involve the foot taiyang/bladder channel will cause back pain, heaviness in the head, cold chills over the spine, then severe fever. When the fever ceases, there is perspiration. This type of malaria is difficult to remedy. One should acupuncture by bloodletting at weizhong (B40).

"Foot shaoyang/gallbladder malarial conditions cause extreme fatigue. The chills and fever are not as severe, but there is an aversion to people; in fact, people frighten the patient. The fever lasts longer than the chills. There is also profuse sweating. One should acupuncture points on the foot shaoyang.

"In foot yangming/stomach malaria there is initially an aversion to cold that is followed by severe chills. The chills last longer, and then fever arrives. When the fever recedes, one will perspire. The patient is attracted to light and warmth, which give temporary relief. One should needle chongyang (ST42).

"In foot taiyin/spleen malaria the patient has fullness of the chest, depression, sighing, lack of appetite, alternating chills and fever, and profuse sweating. During acute attacks the patient is likely to vomit, which provides relief. One should needle points on the foot taiyin channel.

"In foot shaoyin/gallbladder malaria the patient will exhibit severe projectile vomiting, alternating chills and fever with the fever more severe than the chills, aversion to wind, and a preference to seal the windows and doors. This is a difficult condition to treat.

"In foot jueyin/liver malaria conditions the patient will experience back pain, lower abdominal distension, dysuria, frequent but difficult urination, fear, and fright. One should needle points on the foot jueyin channel.

"In lung malaria, the patient feels severe anxiety, and cold so severe that it turns into fever. Needle the hand taiyin/lung and hand yangming/large intestine channels.

"In heart malaria the patient feels restless and hot, with a desire for cold water; chills which are more severe than fever. One should needle the hand shaoyin/heart channel.

"In Liver malaria the patient shows a blue-green hue in the face. The attack is so severe that the patient appears to be dying. Needle the foot jeuyin/liver channel and use bloodletting.

"In spleen malaria the patient experiences chills and abdominal pain. There is borborygmus and severe perspiration. Use foot taiyin/spleen points when acupuncturing.

"In kidney malaria the patient demonstrates a frozen cold appearance. There is severe back pain, difficult movement, constipation, vertigo, blurry vision, and cold extremities. Acupuncture foot shaoyin/kidney and foot taiyang/bladder points.

"In stomach malaria the patient feels very hungry just before an attack, but cannot eat. After eating there is great fullness and distension. Acupuncture points on the foot yangming/stomach and foot taiyin/spleen channels, especially performing bloodletting on the luo points.

"In the treatment of malaria, one must treat just before the attack of fever. One should puncture the artery on the surface of the foot and perform bloodletting. This will immediately reduce the fever. One should also treat just before the chills by acupuncturing hand yangming/large intestine, hand taiyin/lung, foot yangming/stomach, and foot taiyin/spleen points. If the patient's pulse is full, large, and rapid, one should acupuncture the back shu points of all the zang organs. Prick to bleed pohu (B42), shentang (B44), hunmen (B47), yishe (B49) and zhishi (B52). If the pulse is strong but small and rapid, one should moxa points on the foot shaoyin channel. Acupuncture the jing/well points on the tips of the toes. If the pulse is large, slow, and deficient, one should use herbs but not acupuncture.

"Generally speaking, in the treatment of malaria, one should treat thirty minutes before the attack. If this time is missed the opportunity is lost. When no pulse is detected in malaria, one should immediately perform bloodletting on the jing/well points on the tips of the fingers. This will resuscitate the patient. Prior to treatment, look for small red bumps whereupon acupuncture can be performed.

"We have described twelve different malaria conditions. They vary in their manifestations and times of attack. One must observe the patient very closely to determine which type is present. This is the only way to grasp the opportunity of treatment. One can expect results after one treatment; after two treatments the condition will substantially improve; by the third treatment the problem can be cured. If no cure has occurred, bloodletting of the arteries underneath the tongue at lianquan (extra point) can be utilized. If this is still ineffective, perform bloodletting at weizhong (B40). Also use the back shu/transport points below the neck such as dashu (B11) and fengmen (B12). This will surely produce results.

"The physician must always determine precisely the location of the initial symptoms during attacks. Focus the treatment in that area first. For example, if the condition begins with headaches and heavy-headedness, one should prick points of the head and cheek, and between the eyebrows. If it is in the neck and upper back area, use local points again. If it is in the lower back, use weizhong (B40) to let blood out. If in the arms, use points such as shaochong (H9) on hand shaoyin and shangyang (LI1) on the hand yangming/large intestine channels. If in the feet, acupuncture lidui (ST45) on the tip of the third toe along the foot yangming/stomach channel.

"Malaria beginning with sweating and aversion to draft is called wind malaria. Perform bloodletting on the back shu/transport points of the yang channels. If the calves are very sore to the touch, a condition called fu shui bing or marrow-deep pathogen, perform bloodletting at yangfu (G38). This can help stop the pain. If the patient feels mild body ache, use points on the spleen channel. One must be careful, when acupuncturing the jing/ well points of the yin channels, not to let blood out. One should treat every other day. For malaria conditions that attack every other day and that are not accompanied by thirst, acupuncture points on the foot taiyang/ bladder. If there is thirst, acupuncture foot shaoyang/gallbladder points. In febrile malaria with no sweat, use the 59-point method."*

---

*See chapter 61 for a listing and discussion of the points.

CHAPTER 37

PATHOLOGIC DISORDERS OF
HEAT AND COLD

HUANG DI asked, "How do heat and cold transfer among the five zang and six fu organs?"

Qi Bo answered, "Cold will move from the kidneys to the spleen. In this case, one will manifest edema and swelling and deficiency of qi. Cold will then transfer from the spleen to the liver. One will manifest swelling and spasms of the tendons. Cold will then transfer from the liver to the heart. One will become confused and experience obstruction of the chest. Cold will then transfer from the heart to the lungs. One will manifest exhaustion and insatiable thirst. This is called fei xiao, or lung exhaustion, and for every part of water consumed, two parts will be excreted. This eventually leads to death by dehydration. When cold moves from the lungs to the kidneys, one will manifest significant swelling of the abdomen, as in ascites, with gurgling sounds.

"When heat transfers from the spleen to the liver, one will manifest anxiety, fearfulness, and epistaxis. When heat transfers from the liver to the heart, the result is death. When heat transfers from the heart to the lungs, one will manifest ge xiao, diaphragm exhaustion. This is a condition of dehydration. When heat transfers from the lungs to the kidneys, one will manifest rou chi or convulsions, a condition of stiffness and immobility of the spine. When heat moves from the kidneys to the spleen, it depletes and drains the spleen. If one contracts dysentery, it may result in death. When pericardium heat transfers to the bladder, one will have dysuria and hematuria. When bladder heat transfers to the small intestine, it causes constipation. This heat rises, causing ulcerations of the mouth. When small intestine heat transfers to the large intestine, fu jia, or mass in the colon, is the result. Hemorrhoids can also occur. When large intestine heat moves to the stomach, it causes a great increase in appetite, with loss of weight and strength. When stomach heat transfers to the gallbladder, the results are similar to stomach heat. Gallbladder heat moving to the brain causes sinusitis with burning of the sinuses and constant drainage, some bleeding, and blurry, tearing eyes.

"The above conditions are all due to the abnormal transference of pathogenic qi, pathogenic heat, and cold throughout the zang fu system."

CHAPTER 38

ETIOLOGY, DIAGNOSIS, AND TREATMENT OF COUGH

—

H UANG DI said, "When the lungs are diseased, one coughs. Why?"
Qi Bo answered, "When any of the five zang and six fu organs are imbalanced, one can begin to cough. It is not limited to the lungs."

Huang Di asked, "Can you explain to me the various types of cough and their pathophysiologies?"

Qi Bo replied, "The skin and body hair are external manifestations of the lungs. These are the first line of defense against pathogens. When a pathogen invades and causes a stagnation of the wei/defensive qi, which flows under the skin, this will affect the lung function of dispersing. It is the failure of the lungs to disperse that causes the coughing. A diet abundant in cold or raw foods will also do this, as the coldness causes stagnation of the stomach qi. The cold then rises with ying/nutritive qi and spleen qi to the lung, causing coldness, stagnation, and cough.

"Imbalances of the other zang fu organs that result in cough usually manifest at specific times of the year. This most often has nothing to do with the lung being invaded by external pathogens. Since the human being is so connected with the environment, when the zang organs are attacked by a cold pathogen, a person will manifest illness. If it is mild, one will cough. If it is stronger and the cold pathogen enters internally, one will manifest abdominal pain and diarrhea.

"When cold invades during the autumn, the lung is affected first; in the spring the liver is affected first; in the summer it is the heart; in the late summer it is the spleen; in the winter it is the kidney. In all instances, the cold can transfer to the lungs, causing cough."

Huang Di asked, "How does one differentiate these types of cough?"

Qi Bo answered, "Cough that is due to lung problems is accompanied by dyspnea and occasionally hemoptysis. There is a stuffy nasal sound during breathing. Cough due to heart problems is accompanied by chest pains and constriction of the throat. Cough due to liver problems is accompanied by pain in the hypochondriac area, immobility, and distension or fullness. Cough due to spleen disorders is accompanied by pain under the right ribs that radiates to the shoulder blade. This limits mobility; moving about aggravates the cough. Cough due to kidney disorders comes with back pain; the cough contains phlegm or saliva."

Huang Di asked, "How does one differentiate the coughs of the six fu?"

Qi Bo answered, "If coughing conditions of the five zang organs become chronic, they will transfer to the six fu organs. If spleen cough is prolonged it will transfer to the stomach. This will manifest as nausea, vomiting, or the vomiting of worms. If liver cough is chronic it is passed on to the gallbladder, with coughing and vomiting of bile. If lung cough is chronic it is passed on to the large intestine; this cough brings incontinence of the bowels. If heart cough is chronic it is passed on to the small intestine; this cough brings on flatulence. If kidney cough is chronic it passes on to the bladder; this manifests as urinary incontinence. If these fu organ coughs continue, they may pass on to the sanjiao, the three cavities. This will cause cough with distension, fullness, and lack of appetite. In all coughs, regardless of origin, the pathogen will congeal and accumulate in the stomach. The pathogen will then move through the channels to the lung, causing cough with rebellious qi, facial edema, copious phlegm, and mucus."

Huang Di asked, "What is the treatment method?"

Qi Bo answered, "To treat cough due to disorders of the five zang organs, one must acupuncture the shu/stream and back shu/transport points. To treat cough due to disorders of the fu organs, one must use the lower he/sea points. If swelling occurs, one must determine the causal organ. Then points on that organ's channel are selected."

CHAPTER 39

—

DIFFERENTIATION OF PAIN

—

HUANG DI said, "I have heard that people who are masterful in the natural laws of the universe have insights into the internal aspects of the body. I also know that one who is skilled in ancient healing methods can combine this knowledge with current developments in medicine, and thereby demonstrate a clear and precise understanding of the zang fu viscera and the various functions of the body. Thus, one with these abilities would search for the truth and understand all things in the universe. Will you describe to me cases you have known so I may share your insight and relieve my ignorance?"

Qi Bo replied, "Precisely what would you like to know?"

Huang Di answered, "I would like to understand pain and its causes."

Qi Bo said, "When the qi and blood flowing continuously through the body within the channels are attacked by a cold pathogen, they stagnate. If the cold pathogen attacks outside the channels in the periphery, it will simply decrease the blood flow. When it attacks within the channels, it actually blocks the qi flow and creates pain."

Huang Di said, "Sometimes a person will have abdominal pain that is relieved on its own. Sometimes the pain is persistent. Some pain is aggravated by touch; some is relieved by touch. Some pain does not respond to touch at all. Some abdominal pain radiates to the arms. Some pain begins in the epigastric area and penetrates to the back. Some pain is localized in the hypochondrium and radiates to the lower abdomen. Some abdominal pain radiates to the pelvis, genitals, or buttocks. Some pain is continuous until it forms a mass. Sometimes pain is so acute that it causes unconsciousness. Some pain induces vomiting or diarrhea. Some abdominal pain causes constipation. How can one differentiate these pain conditions?"

Qi Bo answered, "When pathogenic cold invades the periphery of the channels, it causes contraction of the channels. The contraction of the channels creates a ripple effect to the collaterals. This is what causes the pain. When heat is applied or the body's yang qi is summoned, the collaterals relax and the pain is relieved. If the person is repeatedly subjected to the cold pathogen, the pain will return and linger and become chronic.

"When pathogenic cold attacks inside the channels and battles the yang qi of the body, it causes a fullness in the channels. This fullness is what indicates excess. This type of pain is severe and unrelenting. It is this full quality within the channels that makes the patient sensitive to touch.

"When the cold pathogen attacks between the intestines and the stomach, causing the qi and blood to stagnate, the small collaterals will contract and pool and cause pain. In this case, applying pressure in the form of massage will disperse the stagnant qi and blood and give relief. Heat radiates through the hand of the doctor and the yang qi is attracted to the area. The heat and yang qi help disperse the cold stagnation.

"When a cold pathogen attacks deeply and penetrates into the channels of the back, even massage and pressure will have no impact. When cold attacks the chong channel, one of the eight extraordinary channels, it creates abdominal pain that radiates upward and into the arm. This is because the chong/vitality channel begins at guanyuan (REN4) in the abdomen, and rises upward. In this case, the blood flow of the chong channel will stagnate and cause the radiating pain into the arm.

"When cold attacks the channels of the back, causing blood stagnation, the result is anemia. Pain arises as a result of this blood deficiency. The middle of the back is connected with the epigastrium. Thus, the pain in this instance radiates between the two locations.

"When cold invades the jueyin or the liver channel, it causes contracting pain in the hypochondrium and low abdomen. Because the channel also traverses the genital and inner thigh areas, the cold can also cause pain there.

"When the cold lingers between the peritoneum and the small intestine, causing blood stagnation within the collaterals, the blood is unable to move into the larger channels; it thus accumulates and eventually forms a mass.

"When the cold pathogen invades the five zang organs, it causes a stagnation of the qi flow within the five zang organs. Communication between the five zang is blocked or even severed. The yin qi within each organ congeals and becomes exhausted because there is no flow to nourish it. The yang qi cannot penetrate into the organs. Thus, yin and yang separate. When this occurs, the resulting pain engenders unconsciousness.

When the yang qi breaks through and penetrates into the organs, reuniting with the yin, one will awaken.

"When cold attacks the stomach, it causes the stomach qi to rebel upward. Vomiting ensues with the pain. When cold attacks the small intestine, its qi cannot properly constrict; the subsequent release causes diarrhea. If the pathogenic heat is allowed to accumulate in the small intestine because of stagnation, pain results. Additionally, fever, thirst, a ferocious appetite, and hard, dry stool and constipation will occur."

Huang Di said, "These differentiations can be acquired from inquiry. But how does one tell from simple observation?"

Qi Bo answered, "The various zang fu viscera manifest in different portions of the face. Once you determine the coloration and the part of the face that is discolored, you can know which organ is affected. For example, yellow in the sclera of the eyes and red in the forehead are signs of heat in the liver and gallbladder; white in the lips signifies cold in the spleen and stomach; bluish-green or black anywhere on the face signifies pain and stagnation.

Huang Di asked, "What about using the method of palpation?"

Qi Bo answered, "First one must determine the area of the pain. Then one determines the primary pulse. This pulse indicates which jiao or cavity is involved. If one finds this pulse to be strong, full, and vibrant, there is blood stagnation induced by an external pathogen. This is an excess and yang condition. However, if the pulse is sinking, there is a deficiency of qi and blood. This is a yin condition. All these can be detected by palpation."

Huang Di said, "I understand that many diseases come from disharmony of the qi. They often involve emotional disharmony. For example, when one is angry, the qi rises upward; when one is joyous, the qi disperses; when one is sad, the qi becomes exhausted; when one is fearful and frightened, the qi descends; when one is chilled, the qi contracts; when one is hot, the qi escapes; when one is anxious, the qi scatters and becomes chaotic; when one overstrains, the qi depletes; when one worries too much, the qi stagnates. These nine types of qi disharmony will lead to what kinds of illness?"

Qi Bo answered, "Anger, in severe cases, can cause vomiting of blood and dysentery. Joyousness causes the qi to flow and disperse freely, allowing the ying and the wei or nourishing and defensive qi to permeate throughout. Grief and sadness cause the lungs to overexpand and press upward; this creates stagnation in the upper jiao or cavity. Here the ying and wei qi cannot permeate. This causes heat to be produced and retained in the chest. The heat gradually consumes fluids, leading to thirst, excessive appetite, and fatigue. Fright causes the jing/channel qi to descend, creating a stagnation of the lower jiao. This results in bloating. Chilliness causes the qi to contract, creating a containment of the ying/nutritive and wei/defensive qi. Heat causes everything to flow faster; this opens the pores and allows the ying and wei to escape with sweat. Anxiousness and being startled cause the shen or spirit not to be housed. When the shen is not housed, the qi is reckless and chaotic. Overstrain causes shortness of breath, weakness, and sweating, and thus depletion. Overworrying about many things or obsessing about one thing draws too much qi to the spirit; the qi then does not perform its function of dispersing to other parts of the body. This results in congealing or stagnation of the qi."

CHAPTER 40

—

CONDITIONS OF THE ABDOMEN

—

HUANG DI said, "There is a type of abdominal fullness in which the patient consumes food in the morning but by evening is unable to eat. Can you please explain this illness and its treatment?"

Qi Bo replied, "This condition is called gu zhang, or abdominal tympanites due to parasitic infection. One should employ a potent herb wine, which will produce relief in one administration, and complete recovery in a second administration."

Huang Di said, "This condition is known to recur. Why is this?"

Qi Bo answered, "This is because the patient is not careful with his or her diet. Also, even after a treatment that seems complete, the root often remains. As soon as one strays from the right diet, therefore, the pathogen returns to congeal in the abdomen."

Huang Di said, "There is a type of chest and hypochondriac distension which causes interference to yin. When the condition is acute, one will vomit blood and clear fluids after smelling anything fleshy or fishy. Gradually the extremities become cold; vertigo and dizziness occur, and blood is found in the bowels and urine. What is the cause of this condition?"

Qi Bo answered, "This condition is called xue ku, or withering of the blood. Often it is rooted when one is young and having encountered massive loss of blood. It is also caused by indulgent and excessive sex following drunkenness, which exhausts the jing/essence and damages the liver. In women, amenorrhea is often the result."

Huang Di asked, "How do you treat this and achieve a full recovery?"

Qi Bo answered, "One would use four-tenths of a qian* of hai piao xiao (*Os Sepiellaeseu sepiae*) and one-tenth of a qian of qian cao (*Rx Rubia cordifolia*). Blend the two together and roll them into pills with sparrow

---

*Qian is the standard measurement in Chinese pharmacology. One qian is equal to 3.3 grams.

eggs. The pills should be the size of an adzuki bean. Take five pills before meals with fish soup. This will rejuvenate the damaged liver and keep the intestines open."

Huang Di inquired, "There is a condition that involves fullness and hardness in the lower abdomen, where one can actually feel the extent of the mass. What is this condition, and is it treatable?"

Qi Bo answered, "This is called fu liang, or hidden mass. It is caused by pus and blood accumulating in the low abdomen, outside of both the intestines and the stomach. This condition is incurable. In diagnosis, be very careful not to palpate too hard, because rupture can cause instant death."

Huang Di asked, "Why is this?"

Qi Bo replied, "The strong pressure causes the pus and blood to exude through the urethra or anus, or it can force the contents upward between the epigastrium and diaphragm, forming a boil. If this condition is above the umbilicus it is terminal; if below the umbilicus the prognosis is slightly better. But in neither case can you palpate harshly. I have discussed this in our talks on acupuncture."

Huang Di asked, "What condition is it when someone suffers from swelling in the major joints and also has pain around the navel?"

Qi Bo said, "This is also fu liang. This occurs because one is invaded by wind cold during sleep. The wind cold permeates the large intestine, causing the intestines to wrap around the navel. There is excruciating pain, and one should not use purgatives. If one mistakenly uses these herbs, obstruction of urine will result."

Huang Di said, "You mentioned previously that in febrile disease or diabetic exhaustion, one should not consume fatty, sweet, or rich foods; the doctor should not use aromatic herbs or heavy minerals. Fragrant herbs can cause manic reactions, and heavy minerals can cause epilepsy. The typical patients who suffer from these two conditions are often wealthy. You ask them to refrain from a rich diet, which they may resist; yet you also do not use expensive aromatic and mineral herbs. How do you proceed then?"

Qi Bo answered, "Aromatic herbs may be too dispersing. The dispersing can cause the pathogen to enter the orifices. Heavy minerals are too strong and have a rapid-acting and harsh quality. Unless the patient is of a calm nature, one should not prescribe these herbs."

Huang Di asked, "Can you explain this further?"

Qi Bo replied, "Heat conditions are already harsh. The use of harsh herbs will injure the spleen qi. The spleen is the earth and disdains domination by wood. The use of these herbs on jia yi days will surely cause the condition to worsen."

Huang Di said, "There is a condition that involves pain and swelling in the neck, coupled with fullness or distension of the chest and abdomen. What is the cause of this condition and how is it treated?"

Qi Bo answered, "This condition is called jueni or extreme cold and morbid condition. If one uses moxa, there may be loss of voice. If one uses acupuncture, the patient may become manic. You must wait, therefore, until the yin and yang qi come together to harmonize. Then treatment may begin."

Huang Di asked, "Why is this?"

Qi Bo replied, "This condition is marked by an excess flow of yang qi upward, which stagnates in the upper jiao. Moxa aggravates the yang condition, which causes it to further dominate the yin. Acupuncture allows this yang qi to escape outward, which causes a disturbance in the shen/ spirit. You must wait for a union of the yang qi and yin qi; the yang qi should descend. Then you may treat and render the cure."

Huang Di asked, "How do you know when a woman is pregnant or suffering from abdominal illness?"

Qi Bo answered, "You should observe the symptoms carefully. The body seems disordered or diseased but the pulses are not pathological."

Huang Di said, "There is a condition that manifests as fever and pain. Can you please explain?"

Qi Bo answered, "All febrile diseases are considered yang and have yang pulses. You must examine the three yang channels of the body at ren ying (ST9). If the pulse at ren ying (ST9) is twice as large as the radial pulse, the condition is in the shaoyang stage. If the pulse at ren ying (ST9) is three times as large as the radial pulse, the condition is in the taiyang stage; if four times as large and full, the condition is in yangming. As the condition progresses into a yin stage, the head and abdomen are affected. One then sees pain in the head and abdominal pain or distension."

CHAPTER 41

—

ACUPUNCTURE IN THE TREATMENT OF BACK PAIN

—

Qi Bo said, "In a condition of the foot taiyang/bladder channel with back pain, the pain will radiate from the neck down the spine. The patient will feel as if carrying a heavy load. One should needle and bleed weizhong (B40). In spring, however, do not let any blood extravasate.

"In a foot shaoyang/gallbladder channel condition of back pain, the pain feels as if one is being needled; there is difficult movement, one cannot arch the back or rotate the head to look backward. In this case one should needle yanglingquan (G34) and let out some blood. During the summer, however, do not allow blood to escape.

"In foot yangming/stomach channel conditions of back pain, the pain is severe; one cannot rotate the head to look backward. If one does look backward, one will experience dizziness and blurry vision. One will also tend to be sad. The physician should needle Zhusanli (ST36) three times to regulate the flow of energy between the upper and lower body. Bloodletting should be performed, although in the autumn this is contraindicated.

"In back pain of foot shaoyin/kidney origin, the pain will radiate along the spine. The physician should needle the point fuliu (K7) on the inner ankle. During spring, bloodletting is contraindicated. If the patient does bleed, the condition will be difficult to cure.

"In back pain of foot jueyin/liver origin, the lower back is very stiff, tense, and arched like a bow about to snap. One should palpate on the inside of the calf muscle above the ankle bone at ligou (LIV5), where there are likely to be soft lumps or nodules. This is where one should needle. If the patient tends to be excessively verbal, or abnormally subdued, the needling should be performed three times.

"In back pain resulting from a disorder of the foot taiyang/bladder channel, sometimes the pain will radiate to the shoulder. There will be blurry vision and bed-wetting. Acupuncture and bleed the dark-colored vein just lateral to weizhong (B40) at the back of the knee until the blood turns from purple to bright red. Pain of a foot taiyang origin in the lower back will make the patient's low back feel as if it is broken. This will cause fear and fright. Acupuncture weiyang (B39), lateral to Weizhong (B40), where the collateral feels like a kernel of corn. Extravasation of very dark blood will occur; stop when the bleeding turns red.

"Disease of the tongyin mai or luo collateral of the foot shaoyang channel that results in back pain makes the patient feel as if being hit with a hammer. This causes the tendons or soft tissue to suddenly swell up. In this case, acupuncture the foot shaoyang channel at yangfu (G38) three times.

"Back pain due to disorders of the yangwei/yang-regulating channel causes sudden swelling, too. When acupuncturing points on this channel, one finds a convergence with the foot taiyang channel in the calf area. Needling thus takes place at chengshan (B57).

"Disease of the dai/belt channel causing back pain results in the patient's being unable to arch the back. If an attempt is made to do so, the patient will fall down. This disease is usually induced by lifting something heavy, which causes the horizontal collaterals to become obstructed with blood. In this case, needle weiyang (B39) and yinmen (B37) twice each, allowing blood to escape.

"Disease of the ren/conception channel that causes back pain results in perspiration; when this stops, one experiences thirst with desire to drink, but afterward one will have discomfort resting. Acupuncture chengjin (B56) three times.

"Disease of the foot taiyang causing back pain manifests in sudden swelling and inflammation of the tendons and ligaments. This is accompanied by grief or terror. Acupuncture the converging points of the foot taiyang and foot shaoyin channels at zhubin (K9).

"Disease of the foot shaoyin resulting in back pain manifests with pain radiating to the chest area; blurry vision also results. In severe cases, the back cannot be straightened and the tongue is contracted. There is difficulty speaking. In such a case, acupuncture jiaoxin (K8). This connects to the yinqiao/yin heel channel points.

"Back pain from disease of the luo channel of the foot taiyin/spleen results in fever; if severe, irritability or delirium result. There may be bed-wetting. Below the waist the sensation is like a broken piece of wood poking the lower back. Acupuncture diji (SP8) three times in the inside knee area between the bone and flesh where you can see several tendons.

"Back pain from disease of the foot shaoyang results in pain so severe that if one coughs, the tendons of the entire body will go into spasm. Acupuncture yangfu (G38) two times.

"When back pain radiates to the spine and up to the neck, causing stiffness, blurry vision, and dizziness, one should acupuncture weizhong (B40) on the foot taiyang and let out blood. When back pain is accompanied by chills, one should acupuncture the foot taiyang and foot yangming channels. If back pain is accompanied by fever, one should acupuncture the foot jueyin channel. If the patient cannot lie flat, one should needle the foot shaoyang channel. If there is fever and dyspnea, needle the foot shaoyin channel; also perform bloodletting weizhong (B40). When back pain is accompanied by chills in the upper body with a stiff neck, pain, and inability to rotate the head, one should acupuncture the foot yangming channel. If there is fever in the upper body, one should needle the foot taiyin channel. If the pain is accompanied by fever and dyspnea, needle the foot shaoyin. If there is also constipation, needle foot shaoyin points. If there is abdominal distension and fullness, needle the foot jueyin. If the back feels broken and the patient cannot lie flat or move about, needle the foot taiyang. If the pain radiates along the vertebrae, needle the foot shaoyin channel. If the pain radiates to the lower abdomen and there is difficulty lying on the back, needle the lower baliao points, which are eight points on the foot taiyang/bladder channel located in the sacral foramen.

"When treating back pain with acupuncture, the number of treatments required should follow the lunar calendar. Generally, in the period of the waxing moon the treatment frequency increases while in that of the waning moon the frequency decreases. For instance, on the fourth day starting from the new moon, perform acupuncture four times; on the fifteenth day after the full moon, acupuncture fifteen times. On the sixteenth day, needle fourteen times; on the twentieth day, needle ten times. Additionally, use the principle of opposite side treatment by treating the left side pain with the points on the right, and vice versa.

"The result from following this principle is often immediate pain relief."

CHAPTER 42

—

THE PATHOLOGY OF WIND

—

HUANG DI stated, "When wind attacks the body, some will manifest with fever and chills, some with fever only, and some with chills only. In some cases this will manifest with li feng, or leprosy, and some with pian ku, or hemiplegia. Some will manifest with wind disease. The cause is the same, but the pathological manifestations are different. Sometimes the pathogen penetrates deep into the interior and damages the zang fu viscera. I do not completely understand the mechanisms of this."

Qi Bo answered, "When wind attacks the body at the superficial level of the skin and prevents the interior from communicating with the external channels, when the body cannot disperse at the superficial level, or when wind exhibits its characteristics of speed and rapid change, chills are the result. Chills also result from the pores being kept open. Conversely, when the pores are closed, one becomes stuffy and feverish. When one is cold, there is a decrease in appetite; when one is feverish, one suffers emaciation of the muscles.

"When wind travels from the yangming/stomach channel into the stomach, it then follows the channel up to the eyes. In an obese person, the wind cannot escape, and lingers. Heat builds up, causing fever, and there is yellowing of the eyes. In a thin person, the yang qi disperses outward. This, of course, causes a feeling of cold. The eyes then display a constant tearing.

"When wind enters the body in the taiyang/bladder channel and scatters in the flesh, a battle with the wei/defensive qi ensues. Obstruction in the channel results, with swelling of the muscles, or boils and carbuncles. This is a result of the stagnation of wei qi. Tingling and numbness often occur. The li feng condition occurs when wind attacks the channels and causes the ying/nutritive qi to heat up. The ying qi becomes degenerative and the blood becomes turbid, spreading toxins throughout. The septum gets inflamed, the skin inside the nose ulcerates, and lesions develop. All began from invasion of wind cold and its lingering aftermath in the channels.

"The season of spring and the days of jia yi belong to the wood element. If one is careless, one can be attacked by wind; this is called liver wind. Summer season and bing ding days are fire. If one is attacked by wind at these times, it is known as heart wind. Late summer and wu ji days are earth; here an attack of wind is known as spleen wind. Autumn and gen xin days are metal; an attack of wind is known as lung wind. Winter and ren quai are water; an attack of wind is called kidney wind. When wind attacks the zang fu viscer shu/stream points and penetrates deeply, it is known as zang fu wind. Wind is able to penetrate because of weakness and deficiency in the body. Typically, the body is weak on one side or at one point. This is called pien feng, one-sided wind.

"When the wind attacks and enters fengfu (DU16), it follows the channel upward to the brain. This is known as nao feng or brain wind. When wind penetrates the head via the eyes, it is known as mu feng. The eyes then feel an aversion to wind and coldness. When wind attacks one who has been drinking alcohol, it is known as lo feng. When one sweats during sex, and then is attacked by wind, this is known as nei feng. Attack by wind after washing the hair is known as tou feng. When wind lingers at the flesh level and progresses into the intestines, causing diarrhea, we call this chong feng. When wind is between interior and exterior and there is spontaneous sweating, we call it xie feng.

"You can see that wind is the cause of many illnesses. Once it penetrates the body, its nature is dynamic and changeable, and it has many pathological manifestations. But the cause is always the same: pathogenic wind attacking the body."

Huang Di asked, "Can you teach me what the signs and symptoms of each zang organ wind are? What are their differentiations and diagnostic keys?"

Qi Bo replied, "Lung wind often causes an aversion to wind, with spontaneous sweating. The face is pale and there may be cough and shortness of breath. During the day, the condition is milder; at night it worsens. There is paleness above the eyebrows.

"Heart wind manifests with aversion to wind and excess sweating. There is dryness and cracking of the lips and tongue. Body fluids are depleted. The patient has a red face and angers easily. In severe heart wind, the speech is slurred. One should look for bright redness in the mouth or lips.

"Liver wind causes profuse sweating and an aversion to wind. Sadness and grief manifest; there is a slight greenish-blue in the face, dryness of the throat, and the patient is easily angered. There may be a dislike of provocative people. One should look for a green-blue color under the eyes.

"Spleen wind manifests with excess sweating, aversion to wind, tiredness, heavy limbs, a dull yellow face color, and a lack of appetite. There is a yellowing, especially of the nose.

"Kidney wind manifests as excess sweating and aversion to wind. There is a dull gray cast to the face and swelling of the eyes. The face may even have a charcoal hue. There is back pain and an inability to straighten. There may be obstruction of the urinary tract. One should look for a dark black color or hue in the flesh.

"In stomach wind, there is excess sweating of the neck, an aversion to wind, lack of appetite, stagnation of the epigastrium and diaphragm, and abdominal distension. Consuming cold foods causes diarrhea. There may be emaciation of the body except for the abdomen, which is distended.

"In tou feng, wind of the head, excess sweating occurs in the head and face. There is aversion to draft. On the day before the weather changes, a severe headache will occur. The patient cannot go outside. On a windy day, the pain actually decreases.

"In lo feng, there is intermittent excessive sweating and aversion to draft. Sweating follows eating. In severe lo feng, the patient is always drenched with perspiration. There is a dry mouth, thirst, and lack of stamina.

"In xie feng there is excessive sweating, dry mouth, and moist skin. There is a lack of stamina along with body aches and chills."

Huang Di replied, "Thank you."

CHAPTER 43

—

THE BI SYNDROME

—

Huang Di asked, "How does bi, or arthralgia condition, come about?"

Qui Bo answered, "A combination of three pathogens—wind, cold, and damp—invades the body, leading to obstruction and causing bi. When wind predominates, we call it xing bi, or moving bi; when cold predominates, we call it tong bi, or painful bi; when damp predominates we call it zuo bi, or tenacious bi.

Huang Di asked, "How is the bi condition further differentiated into five types?"

Qi Bo answered, "In this differentiation, we primarily discuss location. In winter it is termed gu bi; gu means bones. In spring it is termed jin bi; jin means tendons. In summer it is termed mai bi; mai refers to the pulses or channels. In late summer it is termed ji bi; ji means flesh. In autumn it is termed pi bi; pi means skin."

Huang Di said, "I have heard that in the bi condition, the pathogen can attack the internal viscera and stagnate within. How does this come about?"

Qi Bo replied, "The five zang organs are connected externally with their corresponding channels. When the pathogen lingers on the surface, it gradually seeps into the internal organs. If the gu bi lingers and the patient is reinvaded by the pathogen, the pathogen will then attack the kidneys. If jin bi lingers, it will eventually attack the liver. If mai bi lingers, it will attack the heart. If ji bi lingers, it attacks the spleen. If pi bi lingers, it attacks the lungs. Thus, various bi conditions attack during various seasons, affecting both specific parts of the body and then the internal organs.

"As the different organs are attacked, different conditions manifest. For example, lung bi manifests as restlessness, irritability, and fullness of the chest. This is coupled with dyspnea and vomiting. Heart bi manifests as obstruction of blood vessels, irritability, pulsation of the epigastrium, dyspnea, dryness of the throat, sighing, and fright. Liver bi manifests as anxiety during sleep, waking up startled, frequent thirst and urination, pain radiating from the ribs to the low abdomen. The abdomen swells, as if one is pregnant. Kidney bi manifests as distended abdomen, weak bones, difficulty walking or not being able to walk at all. The body is contracted and unable to straighten; in fact, the spine is higher than the head. Spleen bi condition manifests with tiredness and lack of strength in the extremities, cough, vomiting of clear fluids, and obstruction above the diaphragm. Bi of the intestines, chong bi, manifests as frequent thirst, difficulty urinating, borborygmus. The yang qi of the stomach and intestines battles with the pathogenic qi; there is diarrhea with undigested food. Bi of the bladder manifests with tenderness of the low abdomen. There is burning urination, and the bladder feels as if it is filled with hot soup; there is also clear nasal discharge.

"When all is orderly, the individual spirits of the five zang organs are held and nurtured properly. When there is disorder, these spirits disperse or are lost. When one overeats, the stomach and intestines are damaged. When breathing is rapid and difficult, the pathogen has invaded and caused bi of the lungs. When one overworries, the pathogen has affected the heart, causing bi. Bed-wetting is a result of kidney bi. Extreme exhaustion demonstrates that the bi is in the liver. Emaciation of flesh is caused by spleen bi. The various kinds of bi are difficult to cure. They tend to linger, and often begin in the exterior before migrating inward. The bi conditions that are due predominantly to wind have a better prognosis."

Huang Di asked, "Some people, when contracting bi, suffer from chronic pain. Some are cured very quickly, and yet some become very sick and lead to eventual death. Why is there this disparity?"

Qi Bo answered, "When bi conditions penetrate to the five zang organs, death will result. When bi lingers in the bones and tendons, it remains for a long time. When bi lingers in the skin and muscles, it is easily resolved."

Huang Di asked, "What occurs when bi attacks the six fu organs?"

Qi Bo replied, "This is usually due to diet. There can also be attack from the exterior. The six fu have their corresponding shu points, and wind, cold, or damp can invade there and cause digestive problems. This invasion can also combine with dietary factors."

Huang Di asked, "How do you utilize acupuncture in treating bi syndromes?"

Qi Bo answered, "For the five zang, access the shu points; for the six fu, access the he/sea points. Follow the channels that are affected and treat their corresponding points."

Huang Di said, "Can ying qi and wei qi stagnate and cause bi?"

Qi Bo replied, "The ying is the essence extracted from food. It is transported through the six fu via the actions of the five zang, through the channels, and finally nourishes the zang and connects with the fu. The wei is the defensive qi that is formed from the same foodstuff; this qi is different; it is fast and smooth. It cannot travel within the blood vessels but flows between the skin and muscles. It circulates through the chest and remains outside of the channels and vessels.

"If the ying and wei lose their orderly flow, one will suffer from imbalance and disease. However, all one needs to do is restore the orderly flow again and illness will be resolved. If the ying qi and wei qi do not combine with wind, damp, or cold, bi conditions will not occur."

Huang Di asked, "Some bi conditions are painful, while others are not. Some cause numbness, chills, fever, dry skin, or clammy skin. What is the reason for this?"

Qi Bo replied, "If there is pain, cold is dominant. If there is no pain but there is numbness, the condition is chronic; the pathogen has penetrated to obstruct the flow of ying and wei, and the channels have become empty. There is thus no sensation in the skin, because of lack of nourishment and protection. When dryness dominates, the ying and wei are obstructed and do not nourish the skin. If one feels chilled, yang qi is deficient and yin qi is in excess. If one feels feverish, yang is abundant and yin is insufficient. When damp dominates, one is clammy or moist."

Huang Di asked, "What occurs in a bi condition that is not painful?"

Qi Bo answered, "When bi is in the bones, the body feels heavy. When bi is in the blood vessels, the blood will not flow properly. When bi is in the tendons, one is contracted and cannot straighten. When bi is in the muscles and flesh, one feels numb. When bi is in the skin, one will feel chilled. In these conditions, one does not necessarily feel pain. Generally, bi conditions exposed to cold result in acute flareups, while bi exposed to heat decreases in intensity."

CHAPTER 44

—

WEI CONDITIONS

—

HUANG DI asked, "How is it that disorder of any of the five zang organs can cause a wei or flaccidity condition?"

Qi Bo answered, "The lungs govern the skin and body hair. When the lungs are attacked by a heat pathogen, exhausting body fluids, the lobes of the lungs become atrophied—a dry wei condition. The skin and body hair become cracked and brittle. When the heat lingers chronically, paralysis of the extremities results.

"The heart is responsible for blood flow. When the heart is attacked by heat, the blood flows upward. This creates a condition of excess in the upper and deficiency in the lower. The deficiency below produces hollow vessels and a lack of circulation to the joints. The joints then become stiff. The tendons of the feet become loose and flaccid and the patient is unable to walk.

"The liver governs the tendons and ligaments of the body. When heat attacks the liver, it causes the bile to flow upward, causing a bitter taste in the mouth. The tendons dry up leading to contracture and atrophy, which is a wei condition of the tendons.

"The spleen governs the flesh and muscles of the body. When heat attacks the spleen, thirst, lack of body fluids, and numbness of the muscles and flesh result.

"The kidney governs bone and bone marrow. When the kidney is attacked by heat, the jing/essence is exhausted and the marrow decreases. This leads to dry bones and weakness of the spine. The back becomes so weak that the patient cannot support himself in an upright position. This is a wei condition of the bones."

Huang Di asked, "How does a wei condition happen?"

Qi Bo answered, "It starts in the lungs. The lungs are the highest organs of the body and therefore are a distribution center. It has an intimate relationship with the heart. If the lung is dysfunctional, it leads to wei conditions of the extremities, because it cannot distribute nutrients and qi.

"When one is excessively sad, this damages the pericardium. Heart qi cannot then flow freely. The result is a reckless movement of yang qi, causing extravasation of blood, which accumulates in the lower cavity. This leads to blood in the urine.

"According to the ancient medical classic Ben Bing [Origins of Disease] when the large channels are empty, muscle bi results. This ultimately leads to atrophy of the channels as well.

"When one overindulges in thinking, experiences frustration from not being able to fulfill one's wishes, or overindulges in sex, a man will experience the wei condition of zhong jin or reproductive ligament. This is impotence. In women, this results in leukorrhea. According to the Xia Jing [Classic of Medicine], this condition of paralysis of the ligament is caused by a liver disorder. It is the result of overindulgence in sex and depletion of the jing/essence.

"If one is exposed to damp pathogens over a period of time, the muscles and flesh will be invaded. This causes numbness, and rou wei or wei condition of the flesh. According to the Xia Jing, this condition is always caused by exposure to environmental dampness.

"Overtiredness from traveling through severe heat leads to thirst. The heat is excessive internally. It may then attack the water organ, or kidney. The kidney cannot balance this fire and thus the jing/essence dries up. The bone and marrow then become withered and unable to support the body weight. The Xia Jing states that gu wei, wei condition of the bones, is due to excess heat attacking the kidney."

Huang Di asked, "How does one differentiate the five wei conditions?"

Qi Bo replied, "When there is heat in the lung, the face becomes pale and the body hair falls off. When the heart is attacked by heat, the face turns red and one can see the capillaries. When the liver is attacked by heat, the face is greenish-blue and the nails become dry and brittle. When the spleen is attacked by heat, the face is yellow and there are muscle twitches. When the kidney is attacked by heat, the face turns black and the teeth age prematurely."

Huang Di said, "According to your discussion of wei conditions, one can treat the affected meridian. But traditional medical texts state that when treating wei conditions, one should target the yangming channels. What is your explanation of this?"

Qi Bo answered, "Yangming is the source of nourishment for all the zang fu viscera. Only with this nourishment can the tendons, bones, and joints be lubricated. The chong/vitality channel is considered the reservoir of the twelve main meridians. It is responsible for the permeability of nutrients throughout the body and into the muscles. It works together with the yangming in this function. The yangming/stomach can be said to be the primary channel that is responsible for this. In its distribution it involves the dai/belt and du/governing channels, too. When the yangming channel is deficient, the tendons will become flaccid. The dai channel cannot integrate all the systems, and paralysis of the feet results."

Huang Di said, "Specifically, how does one treat wei conditions?"

Qi Bo answered, "One must tonify the rong/spring points and promote flow through the shu/stream points. This fortifies the deficient, and restores order to what is rebellious. It does not matter whether it is the tendons, muscles, bones, vessels, or flesh. They each have their specific seasonal advantages as well. The treatment plan must take into account these factors in order to rehabilitate wei conditions."

CHAPTER 45

—

JUE CONDITIONS: THE SEPARATION OF YIN AND YANG

—

Huang Di asked, "In jue or syncope conditions, there are both cold and hot types. How are these caused?"

Qi Bo answered, "When the yang qi collapses downward, this is called cold jue. When the yin qi depletes, it is called heat jue."

Huang Di said, "With heat jue, one has fever, but it begins on the bottom of the feet. Why is this?"

Qi Bo answered, "The yang channels originates from the surface of the five toes. The yin channels converge on the bottom of the feet. In the case of heat jue, the yin qi is exhausted; therefore the dominant heat emanates from the bottom of the feet."

Huang Di asked, "In cold jue, there are severe chills that begin from the five toes and move up toward the knee. What is the reason for this?"

Qi Bo replied, "The yin qi originates on the inside of the five toes. In cold jue, yang qi collapses downward. Because the yang is insufficient, yin becomes the predominant factor and moves up to the knee. This type of cold progression is not typical of an exogenous cold attack, which moves downward. Cold jue instead begins at the bottom and moves up, as a result of internal collapse of yang."

Huang Di asked, "Can you please explain the mechanism underlying cold jue conditions?"

Qi Bo answered, "The genitals are the meeting place for the spleen and stomach channels. In the summer and spring, the yang qi dominates and the yin qi recedes; in the autumn and winter, vice versa. A person must be aware of these natural energetic changes. If in the autumn and winter, when yang qi recedes, one abuses oneself and depletes the kidney jing, subsequently the kidney qi and yang will also become deficient. The result is yang deficiency, which allows the excess yin and cold pathogens to seep upward into the trunk.

"The qi of the zang fu viscera and channels is all derived from the spleen and stomach. With excessive, indulgent, and abusive behavior, coldness will result in the middle jiao. This puts out the digestive fire and interferes with the processes of transformation and transportation. This further depletes the yang qi, causing a condition of yin dominance. The extremities then become very cold."

Huang Di asked, "Can you please explain the causes and mechanisms of heat jue to me?"

Qi Bo replied, "When one drinks wine, the wine enters the stomach. It does not go through the spleen to enter the channels, but rather goes directly through the stomach to the channels and collaterals of the skin. This is why, after drinking wine, the blood flow to the channels and collaterals becomes full. But in the deeper meridians there is an emptiness. The spleen should help the stomach transform and transport jin ye or body fluids, but with overindulgence in wine, the stomach will lack jin ye or body fluids. The spleen, therefore, cannot fulfill its functions. The result is that yin qi is deficient and yang pathogens can enter, causing disharmony of the stomach. A dysfunctional stomach severs the acquired source of nourishment. This affects the quantity of jing/essence and nourishment to the extremities. These patients often abuse themselves with drunkenness immediately after eating, followed by sex. The combination of these activities consecutively creates a depletion of yin qi that allows yang pathogens to converge in the spleen. The wine and food stagnate in the middle jiao; over time, this creates heat. Heat that is excessive in the middle jiao emanates throughout the entire body. Dark urine or blood in the urine results. Wine has a very yang energy, which damages the kidneys, leading to a yin deficiency. The extremities then become feverish and hot."

Huang Di asked, "In jue conditions, some patients manifest extreme swelling and bloating of the abdomen. Some display unconsciousness for up to an entire day. Why is this?"

Qi Bo answered, "When the yin qi is excess in the upper body, there is deficiency in the lower body. This deficiency causes swelling of the abdomen. When the yang qi is excess above and deficient below, the yang qi rising upward causes disruption and chaos. The upper body houses the spirit, and this disruption causes loss of consciousness."

Huang Di said, "I would like to know how the jue condition manifests in each of the six channels."

Qi Bo replied, "In the taiyang channel one would see head swelling and heaviness, inability to walk, dizziness, and fainting. In the yangming channel one would see epilepsy, manic behavior, distension and bloating of the abdomen, insomnia, red face, fever, delirium, and chattering. In the shaoyang channel one would see sudden deafness, swelling of the cheeks, fever, hypochondriac pain, and difficulty in mobilizing the legs. In the taiyin channel one would see abdominal distension and fullness, difficult or incomplete defecation, lack of appetite, vomiting upon eating, and insomnia. In the shaoyin channel one would see a dry mouth, dark reddish urine, abdominal fullness and epigastric or heart pain. In the jueyin channel one would see low abdominal swelling and pain, distension and fullness of the entire abdomen, dysuria, difficulty with bowel movement, preference for curling up, contracting and shrinkage of the testicles and genitals, and a feverish feeling of the thighs. Generally in jue conditions, one should sedate that which is excessive and tonify that which is deficient. This condition is the result of a disorder of each individual channel, and is not affected by disorders of the other channels. There is no transference. One can therefore acupuncture the shu points on the affected channel.

"In a taiyin jue condition there are calf cramps and spasms, and epigastric pain radiating to the abdomen. In this case one should treat points on the affected channel. In a shaoyin jue condition one sees abdominal fullness and distension, vomiting, diarrhea, and watery stools. Again one should treat points on the affected channel. In a jueyin jue condition one sees back pain, spasms, contracture, abdominal fullness, dysuria, and delirium. Again treat the affected channel. If, however, the taiyin, shaoyin, and jueyin channels are simultaneously affected, obstruction of bowels and urine will occur and there will be cold hands and feet. In this case, the patient will not live beyond the third day.

"In a taiyang jue condition one becomes extremely stiff and frozen; there is vomiting of blood and epistaxis. Treat the affected channels. In a shaoyang jue condition there is stiffness in the tendons and joints, an inability to rotate or move the waist area, and stiffness of the neck so that one cannot turn. If the case is complicated by intestinal abscess or appendicitis, it becomes a severe and incurable condition. If accompanied by severe anxiety or being startled, one will die suddenly. In a yangming jue condition one will see dyspnea, cough, fever, timidity, epistaxis, and vomiting of blood.

"In hand taiyin jue, where yin and yang separate, one will see chest and abdominal fullness and cough, and vomiting of clear fluid. Treat the affected channel. In hand shaoyin jue one will see chest pains radiating to the throat accompanied by fever. This is an incurable condition. In hand taiyang jue one will see deafness or loss of hearing, tearing, stiff neck, and stiff back. Treat the affected meridian. When hand yangming and hand shaoyang jue occur together, one will have obstruction of the throat, swelling, and stiffness of the neck. Again, treat the affected channels."

CHAPTER 46

NORMAL AND ABNORMAL COURSES OF ILLNESS

H UANG DI asked, "What kind of method do you use to diagnose patients who suffer from stomach abscess?"

Qi Bo answered, "To diagnose this, you must first palpate the stomach pulse. The pulse will be sinking and thin, indicating that the stomach qi is rebelling upward. When this occurs the carotid pulse is excessive, indicating heat. Because the carotid pulse in the neck corresponds to the stomach, we can detect that heat is trapped in the stomach and cannot disperse. The result is abscess."

Huang Di said, "Thank you for your explanation. People often suffer from insomnia. Can you please tell me why?"

Qi Bo replied, "This is because the zang organs have become affected by emotional difficulties and overfatigue. The patient must recover from the exhaustion before the shen/spirit can become properly nurtured and housed. Sleep will then naturally occur."

Huang Di asked, "What is the reason a patient cannot lie on his back?"

Qi Bo answered, "The lung organ is located at the highest part of the trunk. It acts as an umbrella for the other organs. When the lungs are full of pathogenic qi, the channels and collaterals expand. This affects one's ability to lie flat on the back. This is further expounded in the classic *Qi Heng Yin Yang* [Mysteries of Yin and Yang]."

Huang Di said, "Some people become ill due to rebellious qi. When I examine the patient, I find the pulse on the right hand is deep and tight, while that of the left is floating and slow. How do I find the location of the main diseases?"

Qi Bo replied, "In the winter the right pulse is naturally deep and tight. This corresponds to nature. The floating and slow left pulse is in opposition to the season. This indicates that the kidneys are diseased. The lungs are also involved. Thus, the lower back is painful."

Huang Di inquired, "How do you detect this?"

Qi Bo answered, "The foot shaoyin channel connects with the kidneys and the lungs. When the lung pulse is floating and slow, the indication is that the kidneys are deficient and unable to support the lung pulse. If the kidneys are diseased, the patient manifests back pain."

Huang Di said, "With patients who suffer from abscesses of the neck, one can use acupuncture, moxibustion, and bloodletting. Can you explain the mechanics behind all modalities?"

Qi Bo replied, "In this condition there are different degrees of pathogenic infuence and different conditions. They are all due to the qi stagnating in the neck area. One uses acupuncture to disperse the stagnation. If the abscess is due to qi and blood stagnation, one should utilize bloodletting. This is known as 'same disease but different methods of treatment.' "

Huang Di asked, "How do conditions like mania come about?"

Qi Bo answered, "This is due to yang qi being suddenly stimulated. It has lost its normal direction. The patient manifests an angry disposition, called yang jue, reckless yang."

Huang Di asked, "How do you diagnose this?"

Qi Bo replied, "In healthy people the yangming pulse is distinct. The taiyang and shaoyang channel pulses are not so distinct. When these pulses also become dramatic and rapid, the indication is yang jue."

Huang Di asked, "How do you treat this?"

Qi Bo answered, "Fasting can cure this. When food and drink enter the stomach and intestines, transformation and absorption increase the yang qi. Therefore, cut off the source and recovery will occur. Subsequently, feed the patient a tea made of iron shavings. These have the function of causing the qi to descend and dispersing knots."

Huang Di said, "Thank you. What kind of illness is it when one feels fever, tiredness, profuse sweating like a shower, aversion to wind and drafts, shortness of breath, and difficulty breathing?"

Qi Bo replied, "This is called jiu feng, drunken wind. Use herbs such as ze xie (*Alismatis*) and bai zhu (*Atractylodes*) in amounts of 1 qian or 3 grams each. Combine with an herb called lu xiancao (*Herba pyrola*) in one-half qian. Make them into a powder and take a pinch with the fingers before meals.

Qi Bo digressed so as to quickly add to the earlier discussion of the pulses: "Sometimes one finds the pulse to be thin and small at the deep level, and it feels like a needle. Upon massage, if the pulse will not disperse, it is considered a hard pulse. When the pulse jumps out of the skin, it is called a big pulse."

Qi Bo ended by making reference to the classics: "The ancient classics of medicine spoke of disease. The *Shang Jing* [Classic of Medicine, vol. 1], describes the activities and relationship of the human being to nature. The *Xia Jing* [Classic of Medicine, vol. 2], describes the etiology and pathology of disease. The *Jin Gui* [The Golden Chamber] discusses the diagnosis and prognosis of disease. A fourth classic, the *Ze Du* [Medical Assessment], discusses diagnosing disease through the pulse. Ze means to palpate the pulse, to discern where the disease is located and the mechanism behind it. Du means gathering information from the pulses and merging them with the impact of the four seasons to determine the course of an illness. A fifth Classic, the *Qi Heng* [Extraordinary Illnesses], deals with extraordinary and uncommon illnesses. Diseases that result in death and that are not affected by the four seasons are termed uncommon. Diseases that result in death but that follow the order of the four seasons are considered common."

CHAPTER 47

—

UNUSUAL ILLNESS

—

H UANG DI said, "A pregnant woman, in her ninth month of gesta-
tion, loses her voice. Why is this?"

Qi Bo answered, "The collaterals of the uterus have been pinched by
the fetus."

Huang Di asked, "Why is this relevant?"

Qi Bo replied, "The collaterals of the uterus are connected to the
kidneys. The kidney channel connects to the kidney organs and then travels
upward, ending at the bottom of the tongue. Therefore, when these collaterals are obstructed, the connection up to the tongue is disrupted and
speech is impaired."

Huang Di said, "How do you treat this problem?"

Qi Bo answered, "There is no need to treat this problem. When the
baby is born, the mother shall recover. According to the acupuncture classic
Ci Fa [Acupuncture Techniques], when there is a severe deficiency one
should not utilize acupuncture. Or when there is an overabundance, represented by a fetus growing within the abdomen, one must be careful and
use acupuncture moderately so as not to injure the fetus. Thus, the solution
is the delivery of the fetus."

Huang Di said, "There is a condition where one feels fullness and
distension of the chest and ribs, and rapid dyspnea; this condition can per-
petuate for two or three years. What is it called?"

Qi Bo answered, "This is called xi shi, stagnation of the breath. This
does not cause difficulty with consumption of food or drink. However,
one should not use moxa or acupuncture. The only method of treatment
is Dao-in. This moves the stagnation, then herbs can be used."

Huang Di inquired, "There is also a condition characterized by swelling of the hip and leg. There is a band of pain surrounding the umbilicus.
What is this condition?"

Qi Bo answered, "This is called fu liang or hidden mass. It is due to chronic lingering stagnation of the wind cold pathogen within the body. The pathogenic cold lingers in the intestine below the umbilicus. Thus, one feels pain around the umbilicus. In this condition do not massage carelessly, as this will obstruct urination."

Huang Di said, "There is also a condition where the patient's chi pulse is moving very rapidly. There is contracture of the muscles and tendons as well. What kind of condition is this?"

Qi Bo answered, "This is called zhen jin or tendomuscular disorder. In this condition, the abdomen becomes acutely distended. If the skin appears dark black or white, the prognosis is poor."

Huang Di stated, "What is the nature of a condition wherein the patient has headaches that continue on and on?"

Qi Bo replied, "Usually this is caused by attack of a strong cold pathogen. The cold penetrates deeply into the bone marrow. Since the brain is an extension of the sea of marrow, the cold travels through the marrow, causing headache and toothache. This is also called jue ni or extreme cold and morbid condition."

Huang Di said, "Some people often have a sweet taste in their mouths. What is the cause of this?"

Qi Bo answered, "This is a condition that is due to the essence of the five flavors spilling upward. It is called pi tan or digestive heat. The stomach receives the food, and the spleen extracts the essence of the food. The spleen should then distribute the essence throughout the body. However, in this case, there is heat in the spleen. This causes the food essence to be detained in the spleen. Since the spleen is connected with the mouth, this essence spills upward. This condition is usually caused by a diet rich in fatty food, which generates internal heat. Indulgence in sweets also weakens the spleen, leading to chest and abdominal fullness. This is known as xiao ke, or diabetic exhaustion. One must use lian cao (*Euphorbiae*) here."

Huang Di asked, "What is the cause of a bitter taste in the mouth that is relieved after treating the gallbladder point yanglingquan (G34)?"

Qi Bo answered, "This condition is called dan tan or gallbladder heat. The patient is usually very indecisive and worries a lot. This suppresses the gallbladder function. Thus the bile, instead of being distributed properly, is excreted upward, causing the bitter taste. One must treat using the front mu/alarm point and the back shu/transport point of the gallbladder. This is discussed in the ancient classic *Yin Yang Shi Er Guan Xian Shi* [The Interaction of the Twelve Yin-Yang Officials]."

Huang Di asked, "What are the name and location of a condition of dysuria with frequent urination, fever, tightness or constriction of the throat, rapid excess carotid pulse, a pushing-up sensation in the diaphragm, and dyspnea, which is an excess condition, and another condition or variation with a thin pulse at the cun position at the wrist, which is a deficient condition?"

Qi Bo replied, "These conditions originate in the taiyin level. Because there is excess heat in the stomach radiating upward, the condition moves to the lung. These are called jue conditions and are incurable.

"This is referred to traditionally as a syndrome of five excesses and two insufficiencies. The five excesses are symptoms of fever, constricted dyspnea and throat, excess carotid pulse, diaphragm obstruction, and dyspnea. The two insufficiencies are frequent urination and a deficient pulse. Essentially they point to a state of excess pathogen and deficient body. One cannot purge or sedate the pathogen for fear of weakening the body, nor can one tonify for it may add to the force of the pathogens."

Huang Di said, "Some people are born with epilepsy. How does this come about?"

Qi Bo answered, "This is considered to be tai bing, which means fetal illness. While the fetus was still in the womb, the mother experienced fright or shock. This caused the qi to move upward and not descend. The jing/essence qi then congealed and was unable to disperse. Thus, the fetus is not properly nourished and is born with a defect."

Huang Di said, "What is the condition where there is swelling of the face and eyes, a large but tense pulse, emaciation, loss of both appetite and desire to drink, and a lack of body aches?"

Qi Bo replied, "This is a kidney condition known as shen feng, or kidney wind. When this type of patient can no longer eat or is anxious and startled, the heart qi fails. Death results."

CHAPTER 48

—

EXTRAORDINARY ILLNESS

—

Qı Bo said, "When one finds the pulses of the liver, kidney, and lung to be full and excess because of stagnation of pathogenic qi, one should expect severe swelling conditions. If the lung pulse feels stagnant and full, the patient will manifest dyspnea and distension in the ribs. If the liver pulse is stagnant and full, the patient will experience distension in the liver area, insomnia, anxiety, and difficult urination. If the kidney pulse is stagnant and full, the patient will have swelling in the feet and lower abdomen; the calves are not the same shape and size, and the swelling can extend up through the thigh and hip, causing difficulty walking. The result of this last condition can be hemiplegia.

"If the heart pulse is full and large, and there is fever, the physician will see spasms of the tendons, convulsions, and seizures. If the liver pulse is small and rapid, there is deficient cold in the liver. The patient will also manifest seizures and spasms. If the liver pulse is rushing, or if it cannot be found because it beats so fast, there will be a sudden loss of voice, probably because of fright. Do not treat, but allow the patient to recover without intervention.

"When the pulses of the kidney, liver, and heart are thready, small, and rapid, and the physician cannot find the pulse on the superficial level, the indication is qi stagnating in the abdomen. In fact, it is likely a tumor of the abdomen. When the liver and kidney pulses are both deep, the indication is water in the abdomen. If both are floating, the indication is wind water. When the liver and kidney pulses are both deficient, this indicates death. If they are both small and wiry, the patient is about to manifest hysteria and anxiety attacks. If the kidney or liver pulse is large, rapid, and deep, the indication is hernia. When the heart pulse is rapid and slippery, there is a hernia of the heart. If the lung pulse is deep, the indication is hernia of the lung.

"When the pulses of the bladder and small intestine are racing, the blood has congealed and formed a tumor. When the spleen and lung pulses are racing, a cold pathogen has accumulated and stagnated to cause hernia. When the heart and kidney pulses are racing, snycope is likely. When the stomach and large intestine pulses are large and rushing, this indicates that the patient has been startled. When the spleen pulse is deep, followed by a tendency to bulge outward, the condition is dysentery. The patient will gradually recover. When the liver pulse is small and slow, the indication is also dysentery. This is still relatively simple to treat. When the kidney pulse is small and deep in a dysentery condition, with blood in the stools, heat in the blood, and fever, the prognosis is poor. For a dysentery condition with blood in the feces caused by compound liver and heart dysfunction, the prognosis should be favorable. In the same condition, if the pulse is small, deep, and choppy, along with high fever, the prognosis is very bad. If the fever continues for seven consecutive days, the patient will die. When the stomach pulse is deep and choppy, or when it is floating and large, and the heart pulse is simultaneously small, rapid, and hard, the indication is that the qi and blood are stagnant and cannot pass through the diaphragm. This will result in hemiplegia. A man will be affected on the left side, a women on the right side. If the speech is not affected, the condition is curable. Recovery will occur in about thirty days. If a man is affected on the right side, or a woman on the left, and in addition there is dysphasia, recovery will not occur for three years. If the patient is under twenty years of age, death will occur within three years. In cases of bleeding and epistaxis, when the pulse is large and there is fever, there is danger of death. If the pulse is floating and hollow, there is probably bleeding or a loss of blood.

"Conditions of sudden unconsciousness will usually result in pulses that are racing. There is likely to be difficulty speaking. If a patient has just been frightened or startled, the pulse will appear to speed up; but after three days it will return to a normal rate.

"If the pulse arrives rapidly and is floating, like the bubbles of boiling water or the waves of a river, and in the course of one full breath there are ten beats or more, the indication is that the jing/essence qi in the twelve channels is on the verge of exhaustion. In ninety days death will ensue. When a pulse comes like fire from kindling, burning forcefully and rapidly, the indication is that the jing qi of the heart is lost. By the end of autumn, when all the wild grass in the fields is wilted, one will die. When the pulse comes like wind blowing away the leaves, the indication is that the jing qi of the liver is exhausted. By the time the autumn leaves fall, one will die.

When the pulse is like guests who come and go without reason, or when it feels congealed, sometimes not detectable and sometimes surprisingly strong, this is because the jing qi of the kidney is depleted. Therefore, one will die by early summer when jujube date tree blossoms fall. When the pulse is like a tiny marble that is made of clay, that is round but not smooth, the indication is that the jing qi of the stomach has been depleted and the patient will die at the end of spring, or the beginning of summer, when the elm tree bark peels. When the pulse is long and hard as if there is an object that spans across the fingers, the jing qi of the gallbladder is depleted. The patient will die at the time of the autumn harvest.

"When the pulse is tight, wiry, and thready, the indication is that the jing qi of the uterus is depleted. The patient will talk incessantly and die at the time when the first frost arrives. If the patient is quiet, however, there is hope. If the pulse feels like paint that has been spilled and is flowing in all directions, the physician can count thirty days until the patient's death. If the pulse feels like a fountain, and there is rising but no falling, a floating quality without strength, the indication is that the jing qi of the taiyang channel has been depleted. There will be rapid dyspnea and shortness of breath; by the time one can taste Chinese chives in the spring, death will occur. If the pulse feels like the old dirt of an abandoned mine, big but deficient, and upon deep pressure it disappears, the indication is that the jing qi of the muscles is depleted. The patient will be ashen. This is similar to a dam breaking and the water flooding. By spring, when the vines begin to grow, when wood is strong and earth is weak, the patient will die. When the pulse feels like the epiglottis, big on top and small on the bottom, and is large on the superficial level, the jing qi of the twelve shu/stream points is depleted. Death will occur when the weather freezes.

"If the pulse feels like an open blade, and at the upper level, feels small and racing and sharp, and upon deep pressure it is large and strong, the indication is stagnant heat in the five zang organs. Cold and heat have combined to attack the kidneys. The patient can lie but cannot sit up. By the first day of spring, when the yang is strong and the yin is deficient, the patient will die. When the pulse comes like a bullet, slippery and small and without root, the indication is that the jing qi of the large intestine has been depleted. The patient will die at the beginning of summer, when the jujube date tree sprouts new leaves; this is when fire is strong and metal is weak. When the pulse is floating and light and soft and deficient, like a flower, the patient will be uncomfortable lying and sitting. The patient will also have a tendency to be very fearful and suspicious, and will move with caution and eavesdrop on what others say. This is because the jing qi of the small intestine is depleted. The approximate time of death will be in deep autumn."

CHAPTER 49

CHANNEL PATHOLOGY IN ACCORDANCE WITH THE ENERGY ALMANAC

—

Q I BO said, "When, in the first month of a Chinese calendar year, the yang qi begins to rise and the cold energy of yin is still prevalent and prevents the yang from taking its usual course, the result is symptoms along the taiyang channel—the first of the yang channels—pain and swelling in the low back and thighs. The month corresponds to ying, as in the energy almanac.

"If a patient leans toward deficiency of yang, he or she will have difficulty walking, because during the first month of a Chinese year the yang qi is pushing the cold qi from the frozen earth. The yang qi deficiency will affect the mobility of the limbs, and this results in a crippling type of condition. The patient will also have headache, stiffness, and pain of the neck that may radiate down the spine. As the yang qi rises in the body, it struggles and causes stagnation. Some patients will experience ringing in the ears because the yang qi is becoming lively, like birds and animals awaking from hibernation. When the yang qi is excessive in this instance, it will cause insanity. The yang converges in the head, while the yin converges in the lower body. Yin and yang separate and cause a condition of upper excess and lower deficiency. If the qi rebels upward, causing deafness, the body has lost its regulating function on the qi level. Some patients will even lose their voices, as the yang qi cannot provide for articulation. When one exhausts oneself through excessive sexual activity, depleting the jing, we may see a condition of jue or syncope that causes aphasia and weak extremities. This is because the kidneys are deficient and the shaoyin channel cannot spread the qi through the four extremities.

"The manifestation of the shaoyang channel is pain in the chest and rib area caused by pathogens, especially those originating in the gallbladder. This condition can affect the heart channel, and occurs in the ninth month of a chinese year. Then the yang qi is about to descend while the yin qi is about to rise. These patients cannot lie on their sides. All things in the universe begin to go into hibernation. This is a time to be quiet and passive. People become affected by having a limited mobility. As the excessive nature in this channel increases, one has difficulty performing physical activity. The nature of vegetation at this time is to wilt; thus, one's yang qi also moves from the surface to the interior, while the yin qi strengthens; the yang qi descends while the yin qi ascends. In people this causes twitching of the feet.

"In pathology of the yangming channel, one will see shivering and chills. The yangming channel corresponds to the fifth month of a chinese year that is represented by the symbol wu in the energy almanac. At this time, yang has reached a peak and yin has just begun. In pathology the yangming channel at this time contains an abundance of yang qi. When the yin qi rises, it creates episodes of shivering. Thus, one encounters swelling of the legs and feet, and weakness of the thigh and hip. Asthma and dyspnea occur, due to water accumulation; the water pathogen follows the rise of yin qi. Chest pain, shortness of breath, and shallow breathing ensue. This can progress to a serious state with a grave outlook. The patient prefers a quiet, tranquil place, and may have a fear of associating with people, may prefer the dark, and may have an aversion to noise, especially that made from wood clapping. The yin and yang qi are battling; water and fire do not mix. The excessive yin nature of this imbalance creates a desire to be isolated in quietude and darkness, dissociated from the world. Patients can also manifest the opposite: hysteria, loud crying, singing, and running around naked. In this instance the yang qi wins the battle and travels through the channel, creating disturbance in the disposition. Headaches, sinus infections, and abdominal swelling may result, as the pathogen in the yangming channel travels through the lou collaterals and enters the taiyin channel.

"In taiyin channel pathology there is a condition involving abdominal distension. It manifests as tremendous bloating, distension and fullness in the abdomen. The reason is that taiyin is considered extreme yin within yin. It corresponds to the eleventh month of a Chinese year, or zi in regard to the energy almanac. In the eleventh month the myriad things of the universe are hibernating and storing; the yang qi within the human body has also gone deep inside. The spleen channel enters the abdomen and the luo of the stomach connects to the spleen. Therefore, if the pathogen lodges within those channels, distension disease results. There is a teaching that says as the pathogen rebels up to the heart, it manifests as bulimia, wherein one vomits after eating. The reason is that the yin qi, being excessive, exudes upward, extending its influence into the stomach channel. Since the luo of the stomach travels up to the heart, this yin qi attacks the heart. Burping, belching, and vomiting after eating result. The stomach is unable to digest excess food; thus, it cannot transport the predominant yin, and an overflow at the top results. As the months progress and the twelfth month arrives, the yin qi peaks and begins a downward cycle. As the yang qi mobilizes, it helps the bowels to open and flow and pass gas. Thus, the condition of distension is cured.

"The shaoyin channel has a pathology of back pain. This is specific to the kidney channel in particular. Back pain that results from kidney weakness or disease is caused by the yang qi being subdued in the tenth month. The yang qi descends and back pain results. One will also manifest asthma and coughing because the yin qi permeates the lower body; the yang qi then floats upward, unrooted. When the qi rebels upward, coughing, nausea, vomiting, dyspnea, and asthma result. One may also experience anxiety and restlessness as well as nervous tension, dizziness, and blurry vision. This is all at a time when yin and yang are changing in nature, like the changing of the guards. This is a pivotal point between living and dying. The frost has begun to appear and the heavy, suppressive energy of autumn has already descended on the earth. All things in nature are affected by the suppression of qi; they weaken or degenerate, then return to their root. Within the human body the yin and the yang qi are competing. As the yang qi begins to lose, one experiences anger and blurred vision. When the yang qi loses its regulating effect, the qi of the shaoyang channel cannot flow smoothly and disperse throughout the body. This stagnates the liver qi. The liver then loses its control and restraint of the emotions, and anger prevails. This condition is called jian jue, a simmering condition. Another manifestation may be that one has tremendous fear, as if running from someone and being afraid of being caught. The yang qi has not completely exhausted itself; it enters deeply within, causing a battle of yin and yang. It feels as if one has committed some kind of crime and is in fear of being apprehended. One may also have an aversion to smells. This is because the digestive function of the stomach is weakened; one loses the appetite and has an aversion to the smell of food. The face appears dark, like dirt. This is because the suppressive energy of autumn disperses the essence of the organs. Some patients will have coughing with blood because the luo channels of the upper body have been damaged. The blood fills the vessels of the chest; thus, nosebleeds can also occur.

"In the pathology of the jueyin channel, hernia in women will cause tremendous lower abdominal swelling and pain. Jueyin corresponds to the third month of a Chinese year, or chen in the energy almanac. This is a time when the yin qi is decreasing and the yang qi is increasing. We consider this yin within yang. The yin pathogen congeals within the body, causing hernia or fullness and distension in the abdomen. One may also have pain in the back or spine, making it impossible to lie in a prone position. This is because in nature, as yang qi rises, things begin to grow; but if cold is not completely gone and there is still frost on the ground, yang qi will be slightly inhibited. One is unable to bend the spine; thus lying on the stomach is difficult. Some patients may display swelling of the bladder or urethra, resulting in dysuria. This is because the yin pathogen is excess and obstructs the jueyin channel. There may also be a dry or burning throat. This is the result of yin and yang battling, causing heat or dryness to rise to the throat."

CHAPTER 50

—

RUDIMENTS OF ACUPUNCTURE

—

Huang Di asked, "Could you please tell me the important principles of acupuncture?"

Qi Bo answered, "In disease one must differentiate between the external and the internal location of the pathogen. In acupuncture there are differentiations of deep or shallow insertion. If the illness is on the biao, or external, level, one should insert superficially; if on the internal level, one should insert more deeply. The location of the illness must be reached; but it is important not to insert too deeply so as to not injure the five zang organs. Inserting too shallowly, however, will not allow the physician to reach the area of illness, and the qi and blood can be disrupted, which allows an opportunity for pathogens to enter. Acupuncture performed without a guiding principle can be dangerous or damaging.

"It is said that illness may be on the hair level, the skin level, the muscle or flesh level, the level of the channels, the tendon level, the bone level, or the marrow level. When treating illness on the hair level with acupuncture, do not damage the skin level, as this will affect the health of the lungs. When the lung function is disrupted, by autumn one may become susceptible to malarial diseases. Gradually this may grow into a fear of chills. If the illness is at the skin level, one must take care not to damage the muscle level so as not to impact the spleen function. If the spleen function is damaged, during the last eighteen days of each season the patient will manifest distension, fullness, and loss of appetite. In illness at the muscle level, needling too deeply will damage the channel level. In this case the heart function will be disrupted; chest pain or angina will manifest by summer. In illness of the channels and vessels, needling too deeply will damage the tendon level. This will impact the liver function; by spring, one will manifest febrile disease or a flaccidity of the ligaments and tendons. In illness of the tendons, needling too deeply will damage the bone level. This will impact the kidney function. In this case, during the winter one will experience back pain and distension of the abdomen. Finally, in illness of the bones, needling too deeply will damage the marrow. The marrow then gradually depletes, causing soreness, tiredness, and weakness in the extremities, leading to disability."

CHAPTER 51

—

NEEDLING DEPTH
IN ACUPUNCTURE

—

H UANG DI asked, "Could you please tell me more about proper needling depth in acupuncture?"

Qi Bo answered, "When needling the bone level, take care not to
injure the tendon level. When needling the tendon level, do not injure the
muscles. When needling the muscles, do not injure the channels and vessels. When needling the channels, do not injure the skin. When needling
the skin, do not injure the flesh or muscles. When needling the muscles,
do not injure the tendons. When needling the tendons, do not injure the
bones."

Huang Di said, "I do not feel I truly understand this."

Qi Bo replied, "What is meant by acupuncturing the bone level but
not injuring the tendons? When needling deeply, do not stop at the level
of the tendons before reaching the bone level. Go all the way in one breath,
or in a series of breaths, depending on your technique. But reach that depth
without removing the needle. When needling to the depth of the tendons,
one can avoid injuring the muscles by inserting past them. This logic follows with each specific level. The needle must go to the proper depth; any
depth other than the correct one will cause undesirable effects."

CHAPTER 52

—

CONTRAINDICATIONS
IN ACUPUNCTURE

—

HUANG DI asked, "Can you advise me on the areas that are contraindicated for acupuncture?"

Qi Bo answered, "Each organ has a vulnerable spot. One must take notice and use the utmost care. The liver qi naturally ascends on the left side. The lung qi descends on the right side. The heart regulates the yang qi that circulates on the exterior. The kidney regulates the yin qi on the interior. The spleen transforms and transports the extracted essence from food and drink. This process feeds the other organs. The stomach receives food while promoting digestion. Above the diaphragm there are the organs that sustain life: the heart and lungs. Bilateral to the seventh thoracic vertebra lies the pericardium. Be very careful when needling near these critical organs. If one follows these contraindications, one will not cause trouble. If one violates them, one will be faced with imminent danger.

"What occurs if the physician accidentally punctures the heart? The patient will die in one day, after sighing and belching. If the physician punctures the liver, the patient will die within five days, after displaying delirium and talking to himself or herself. If the physician punctures the kidney, the patient will die within six days, after much sneezing. If the physician punctures the lung, the patient will die within three days, coughing and choking to death. If the physician punctures the spleen, the patient will die in ten days, after constant swallowing. If the physician punctures the gallbladder, the patient will vomit to death within one and a half days. If the physician accidentally punctures the major artery on the surface of the foot, the patient will bleed to death. When acupuncturing the face, if the physician punctures the arteries near the eyes, blindness will result. If the physician acupunctures too deeply at nao hu point (DU17) in the head, the brain will be injured and death will be immediate. If jinjin and yuye (extra points), under the tongue, are punctured too deeply, bleeding will be continuous and aphasia will result. If the physician accidentally punctures the capillaries in the foot, bruising and local swelling will occur. If the physician punctures weizhong (B40) too deeply, the artery will be injured and the patient will fall down and turn pale. If the physician accidentally punctures qichong (ST30) and injures the artery, blood will congeal within, causing swelling. If the physician punctures too deeply between the vertebrae, injuring the marrow in the spine, the patient will experience back pain and suffer a condition similar to rickets or humpback. If the physician punctures the nipple, causing damage to the breasts, swelling and distension will result, along with ulceration and rotting within. If the physician punctures quepen (ST12) too deeply, the lungs will collapse, resulting in cough, dyspnea and difficulty breathing. If one punctures yuji (LU10) local swelling will result.

"One should refrain from acupuncturing patients who are inebriated, as this will cause chaos to the qi and blood. One should not acupuncture a patient who has just experienced rage or anger, as this will cause the qi to rebel. One should also refrain from acupuncturing when the patient is too tired, right after eating, if the patient is extremely hungry or thirsty, if the patient has just experienced shock, or is frightened or startled. If one acupunctures the points on the inner thigh and accidentally punctures the artery, the patient will bleed to death. If one inappropriately acupunctures shangguan (G3) and injures the blood vessel, abscess may develop in the ear, causing deafness.

"When acupuncturing the knee, if the physician causes fluid to ooze, the patient may become crippled. If the physician injures the blood vessels when acupuncturing points on the hand taiyin channel, the patient may bleed to death. When acupuncturing points on the foot shaoyin channel, if the physician causes bleeding and depletion of kidney qi, dysphasia will result. In acupuncturing the chest, if the lungs are injured, the patient will display asthma, dyspnea, difficulty breathing, and the body will remain in a crouched position. When one acupunctures too deeply in the elbow, qi will congeal, causing a loss of mobility of the arm. If one acupunctures the inner thigh too deeply, three cun below the symphysis pubis, incontinence will result. If one acupunctures the ribs too deeply, cough will result. If one acupunctures the low abdomen too deeply, the bladder will be punctured, causing urine to flow into the abdominal cavity. If one acupunctures the calf too deeply, local swelling will result. If one acupunctures too deeply around the ocular orbit, injury to the channels will result in continuous tearing and possible blindness. If one acupunctures a joint too deeply, fluid will discharge, causing loss of flexibility and use of that joint."

CHAPTER 53

——

PRINCIPLES OF TONIFICATION
AND SEDATION
IN ACUPUNCTURE

——

Huang Di asked, "Will you please explain to me the meaning of deficiency and excess?"

Qi Bo answered, "When there is an abundance of qi within, qi on the exterior will also be abundant. When the exterior is weak, the interior is certainly deficient. These are normal patterns. However, if the opposite is true—that is, if one is deficient inside but appears strong on the exterior, or vice versa, it is considered a sign of disease. A good appetite goes together with strong qi; a meager appetite goes with deficiency. The opposite of this is a deficiency condition manifesting good appetite and vice versa. When the pulse is large and full, there is an abundance of blood. When the pulse is small, thready, and weak, there is not enough blood. These conditions are normal; their opposites indicate abnormality."

Huang Di asked, "Now can you tell me how do the opposite or abnormality appear?"

Qi Bo replied, "When the qi is abundant and strong but the body feels cold, or when the qi is deficient within but the body has fever, this opposes the norm and indicates disease. When one has an abundant appetite but one's vitality is deficient, this is also abnormal. When the qi is excessive but one has no appetite, this is also abnormal. When the pulse appears full but the blood is deficient, or when the pulse appears small and feeble but there is an abundance of blood, these conditions too are abnormal and indicate illness.

"When the qi is excessive and there are chills, the body has been invaded by cold pathogens. When the qi is deficient and there is fever, the body has been attacked by summer heat. When the appetite is large but the vitality is deficient, the cause is either loss of blood or an accumulation of damp in the lower body. When the appetitie is meager but there is an abundance of qi, the pathogen is located in the lung and stomach. When the pulse appears small but blood is abundant, the illness is a heat pathogen in the middle jiao or cavity. When the pulse appears large but there is a lack of blood, one has been invaded by wind. One will then lose one's appetite. These are the reasons for abnormal manifestations and courses of illness.

"Generally speaking, what is excess? It means that the pathogen has invaded the body. What is deficiency? It means the body's antipathogenic qi is depleted. Generally excess conditions relate to heat while deficient conditions relate to cold. When treating excess conditions with acupuncture, upon withdrawing the needle, one should allow the opening to stay open in order to dispel the pathogenic qi. In deficient conditions press with the finger on the opening immediately upon withdrawing the needle so as not to allow antipathogenic qi to exit."

CHAPTER 54

—

THE ART OF ACUPUNCTURE

—

H UANG DI said, "Will you please explain to me the nine different needles? And will you also please discuss the methods of tonification and sedation in excess and in deficiency?"

Qi Bo answered, "When acupuncturing deficient conditions one should elicit heat sensation with the needle. Only when the qi is strong will it be able to produce heat. In treating excess conditions one should elicit a cooling sensation. When the pathogenic qi is weakening one will experience a cooling feeling. When there is stagnation in the blood caused by the accumulation of a pathogen, one should promote bloodletting to rid the bad blood. In withdrawing the needle on patients with an excess condition, withdraw the needle quickly. Allow the hole to remain open in order to disperse the pathogen. In deficiency, withdraw the needle slowly and close the hole to prevent loss of qi.

"What is meant by excess and deficiency? This is defined by the sensation of either warming or cooling under the needle when the qi arrives. The physician must be attentive and observant regarding this event. After differentiating the condition as excess or deficiency, the doctor should be well versed in performing tonification or sedation techniques. If the wrong method is used, either tonifying an excess or sedating a deficiency, one has engaged in a violation of practice. In order to master the techniques one must be able to use the nine needles with equal ease. Each of the nine has a specific indication. In terms of the timing in tonifying or sedating, one must coordinate the technique with the opening and closing of the hole, and the arrival and departure of the qi. When the qi arrives, we call this opening. At this point, one can sedate. When the qi leaves, we call this closing. Now one can tonify.

"The nine needles are of different size, shape, and use. When acupuncturing excess, one must sedate. Insert the needles and await the arrival of yin qi. When one feels a cooling sensation under the needle, remove the needles. In deficiency, one must tonify. After needle insertion, await the arrival of yang qi. When there is a warming sensation, remove the needles. Once you grasp the qi with the needle, be very attentive and listen so as not to lose the opportunity to manipulate the effects. Treat disease according to where it is located; determine whether to insert deeply or shallowly. When the disease is located deep, insert deeply. When the disease is superficial, needle shallowly. Although there is a difference in depth of penetration, the principle of awaiting the qi is the same.

"When acupuncturing, one should be prepared and careful, as if one is facing a deep abyss. Move carefully so as not to fall. In handling the needle, hold it as if holding the tiger—firmly grasped and in control. One needs a calm mind to observe the patient. Concentrate clearly on the patient and do not become scattered. Upon inserting the needle, be accurate and precise. It should not be crooked or miss the target. When the needle enters the body, the physician should observe the patient closely in order to help guide the patient's attention. This allows the qi in the channels to move more easily, and the results are more effective."

Huang Di said, "I've heard that the nine types of needles have a relationship to yin and yang and the four seasonal energies. Can you please explain this so it may be passed on to later generations as a principle of healing?"

Qi Bo answered, "In Taoist cosmology the number one corresponds to heaven; two to earth; three to man; four to the seasons; five to sounds; six to rhythms; seven to the stars; eight to wind; nine to the continents. People have physical form and connect to nature. The various shapes and forms of the nine needles conform to different types of conditions. The skin of human beings envelops and protects the body, just as heaven envelops and protects the myriad things. Muscles are soft, pliable, and calm, just as earth, which contains the myriad things.

"People move about and also sleep. The pulse mirrors this with excess and deficiency. The tendons that strap together the whole body have differing uses at different locations. This is similar to the seasons of the year, which have their unique uses and purposes too.

"People's voices correspond to the five sounds. People's six zang and six fu organs are yin-yang couples, similar to the six rhythms and scales. People's sensory organs and their positions, as well as their teeth, are similar to the positions of the stars. People's breath is like the wind of nature. The nine orifices and three hundred and sixty-five luo collaterals spreading throughout the body are like the rivers and tributaries spreading over the earth; they feed the oceans, which in turn surround the nine continents.

"Therefore, we have the nine needles. The first, called chan zhen, superficially punctures the skin. The second needle, called yuan zhen, does not penetrate but instead massages the acupoints on the flesh and muscles. The third needle, ti zhen, punctures the vessels. The fourth needle, feng zhen, punctures and draws blood from capillaries and small veins. The fifth needle, fei pi zhen, lances the skin to drain pus. The sixth needle, yuan li zhen, punctures the joints for bi conditions. The seventh needle, hao zhen, punctures the acupoints on the flesh. The eighth needle, chang zhen, punctures deep fleshy locations. The ninth needle, da zhen, punctures the abdonmen to relieve edema or masses. Choose these needles wisely for the appropriate occasion.

"People's emotions and minds change often. This is similar to the eight unpredictable winds of nature. People's qi circulates ceaselessly, similar to the constantly regenerating quality of nature.

"The teeth and hair grow. The eyes and ears are alert and acute. The articulation of the voice is hoarse or clear. These all have different functions, but all perform their duties correctly. This is similar to the five sounds and six scales; everything has its order.

"The blood and qi within the body circulate throughout the channels and vessels, balancing yin and yang, just as water in rivers and lakes circulates endlessly. The qi of the liver connects with the eyes, and the eyes are part of the nine orifices."

CHAPTER 55

—

ACUPUNCTURE TECHNIQUES

—

Qi Bo said, "One who is well versed in medicine and healing will, before palpating the pulse, listen and inquire about the patient's complaints. When the illness is in the head, causing severe headaches, one should employ acupuncture to the bone level to alleviate the condition. The depth must be exact so as not to injure the bone, the flesh, or the skin. This is so even though the skin provides the entry and exit for the needle.

"There is a method called yang puncturing. This means inserting one needle directly into the middle of the point, then on both the left and right sides of the point, inserting other needles at diagonal angles to support the first needle. This method can be used to treat either hot or cold conditions.

"When the pathogen penetrates deeply, direct the needle at the appropriate zang organ because of its proximity to the pathogen. To do this, utilize the shu/transport points on the back; these are where the individual zang converges. Acupuncture until either the chills or heat in the abdomen disappears or subsides. One must induce slight bleeding as the needle is withdrawn.

"When treating conditions with pus or swelling, one should needle locally. Observe how deep and large the abscess is before acupuncturing. When the abscess is quite large, one should discharge pus and blood. When dealing with small but deep boils, one should needle deeply and straight, to penetrate the proper depth.

"When there is stagnation in the lower abdomen, one should needle downward, finding areas of the abdomen where there is thicker flesh. Needle at an angle, not straight in, from the upper abdomen toward the lower. One should also needle points alongside the fourth lumbar vertebra and lower; that is, down alongside the sacral foramen. Points along the lower rib area can be used as well. This conducts heat from the upper abdomen to the lower to disperse the stagnation.

"When disease in the low abdomen manifests as pain, constipation, or urinary obstruction, we call it shan or hernia. This is due to exposure to cold. One should needle on both sides of the lower abdomen and in the inguinal area. Also acupuncture the lower back and sacrum. Be generous with the number of points. Induce a heat sensation in the low abdomen to disperse the cold.

"When the condition is in the tendon level, causing spasm or contracture of the four extremities, pain in the joints, and limited mobility, we call it jin bi, bi syndrome of the tendons. Begin by needling directly at the painful location on the tendon itself. Because the tendon connects muscle to bone, be careful not to injure the bones. When the tendon begins to feel warm, this indicates that the condition is improving. When the disease is completely cured, stop acupuncturing.

"When the illness is at the flesh or muscle level and causes pain in the skin and muscles, we call this ji bi. This is due to exposure to cold and damp. One should acupuncture points at the separation between large and small muscles. These are known as big points, such as heju (LI4) or yanggu (SI5). The small points are known as xi/cleft points, such as houxi (SI3) and taixi (K3). Insert deeply and generously until the local area produces heat. Be careful not to injure the bones and tendons. If this does happen, boils or abscesses will be caused. If the physician can obtain heat sensations in all these points, recovery will be absolutely aided.

"When the condition is in the bone level, the patient feels heaviness, difficulty in moving, and deep pain and soreness as if in the marrow. The area affected feels very cold. This is known as gu bi, bi syndrome of the bones. Acupuncture deeply, but do not injure the vessels and flesh. In the passage to the bone level, one must select carefully between the large and small muscle groups. Elicit heat sensations radiating from the bones to speed recovery. Stop treating when the patient is well.

"When the illness occurs in the three yang channels of the hand and foot, producing constantly changing cold or hot conditions in different parts of the body, we call it kuang or mania. Acupuncture using sedation method in order to disperse and sedate the pathogen in the yang channels. After treatment, observe the body. If there is a uniform heat sensation over the body, the patient is cured. In the beginning stages, kuang comes once a year. Left untreated, it will progress and flare up once a month. If still untreated, it will flare up once a week. This is known as dian bing or manic-depressive condition. One should acupuncture both the small and large points in all the channels during the acute phase. If the patient has no symptoms between flareups, needle using tonification or sedation depending on what is needed. Continue until cure has been achieved.

"When wind attacks the body, causing alternating fever and chills, perspiration may happen throughout the day. This can occur in severe conditions that are similar to malaria. Treat the skin level, targeting the channels and collaterals. This will induce even more perspiration. If fever and chills remain despite the diaphoretic treatment, one should acupuncture every third day. By the one-hundredth day, the condition can be totally cured.

"Another condition of severe wind attack causes heaviness throughout the body, especially in the joints, and a gradual loss of the eyebrows. This is called da feng, or disease of severe wind similar to leprosy. Acupuncture the flesh. Induce sweating. Treat this continuously for one hundred days at the muscle level; then acupuncture the marrow level. Induce sweating for another hundred days. After two hundred days the eyebrows will regrow and treatment can be ceased."

CHAPTER 56

—

DERMATOMES OF THE CHANNELS

—

Huang Di said, "I have heard that on the skin there are twelve divisions that correspond to the twelve channels. How does a physician gather clues to the nature and prognosis of an illness by observing the skin dermatomes?"

Qi Bo answered, "In order to understand and grasp the skin dermatomes, one needs to trace the channels as they travel. For example, the luo collaterals of the hand and foot yangming called hai fei, or the door, can actually be observed on the skin. When it is blueish in color, this indicates pain. When black, the indication is bi/obstruction. When yellow or red, it indicates heat. When pale, the indication is cold. If all five colors manifest, cold and heat are present simultaneously. Before the pathogen invades the main channels, we can see it in the luo channels. The luo collaterals are considered yang and float to the surface. The main channels are considered yin because they run relatively deep.

"The luo of the hand and foot shaoyang channel are called shu chi or the crossing guard. We can also see these luo on the surface, along their pathways. If the pathogen is excess, it will certainly be transmitted into the main channel. If it is a yang pathogen it will go directly to the channel. If it is a yin pathogen it will go from the channels into the organs. This principle also holds true for the other channels.

"The luo of the hand and foot taiyang are called quan shu or limited crossing. If the pathogen in these luo is excessive, it will be transferred into the main channel.

"The luo of the hand and foot shaoyin are called shu ru or fleshy crossing. If the pathogen is excessive in these luo, it will also transfer to the main channel. When this occurs, it begins in the luo, progresses into the channel, and then follows the yin channels and culminates in the bones.

"The luo of the hand and foot jueyin are called hai jian or inner gate. If the pathogen is excessive in these luo, it progresses into the main channels.

"The luo of the hand and foot taiyin are called quan zhi or closed gate. If the pathogen is excess in these luo, it will also go into the main channels.

"All disease begins at the skin level. When the pathogen invades the skin, forcing the pores to open, it penetrates and lodges in the luo. When it remains, it will transfer to the main channels. If it is not chased away from this point, it will then enter the fu. Here it accumulates in the stomach and intestines. Initially, when disease attacks the skin, it causes one to shiver. The body hair stands on end. One's pores will open to attempt to disperse the pathogen, but often the pathogen will invade the luo. When the luo is full of the pathogen, and the colors change, the pathogen overflows into the main channels. It will do this only when the qi in the channel is deficient. If the pathogen is allowed to linger between the tendons and the bones, and if it is a predominantly cold pathogen, the result will be pain in the bones and spasms in the tendons. If it is predominantly a heat pathogen, the tendons will become flaccid and useless, the flesh and muscles will atrophy, and the body hair will become dry and brittle."

Huang Di said, "You have described the location of the twelve dermatomes on the skin. But what is the pathophysiology behind this?"

Qi Bo answered, "The skin is where all the luo are contained and spread. When the pathogen attacks the skin, it forces the pores open and initially attacks the luo channels. When these fill up, the pathogen flows into the main channels. When these fill, it flows into the fu organs. One can determine decisively where the disease is by observing the skin and the corresponding dermatomes. When one can see changes but nothing is done, the pathogen has the opportunity to travel to the organs and cause major disease."

CHAPTER 57

—

CHANNELS AND COLLATERALS

—

Huang Di said, "The luo collaterals are more superficial than the main channels,* and display varying degrees of color. Some are green, some are red, some yellow, white, or black. What is the reason for this?"

Qi Bo answered, "The colors of the main channels and branches do not change. But the colors of the collaterals are inconsistent."

Huang Di asked, "What are the colors of the channels that stay constant?"

Qi Bo replied, "The channels of the heart are red, the lung white, the liver green, the spleen yellow, and the kidney black. They each have their individual correspondences to the five elements."

Huang Di said, "Are the luo collaterals the same colors as their corresponding channels?"

Qi Bo answered, "The color of the yin collaterals always correspond. But the yang collaterals change color according to seasonal variations. For example, in the winter and autumn, the cool temperature slows down the flow of the blood and qi. One would then typically see green, blue, or black colors. The summer and spring are warmer, and the heat causes a faster flow of the blood and qi. Thus, one sees yellow and red more often. These are all natural changes of colors. If the body displays all five colors in the collaterals, however, this indicates either extreme cold or extreme heat. This acute change is considered pathological."

---

*Channels, or jing, are the main thoroughfares for energy flow within the body. There are twelve main channels, each corresponding to and connecting with a viscus. Collaterals, or luo, are passageways connecting the main channels and are more superficially located than are the main channels.

CHAPTER 58

—

ACUPUNCTURE POINTS

—

Huang Di asked, "I have heard that there are 365 openings called xue or points in the human body that correspond to the number of days in the year. I am intrigued by their locations. Would you please tell me about them?"

Qi Bo bowed, then replied, "This question is not easy. If not for the sages, who would spend time researching this? I will tell you everything I know to help clarify the locations of these points."

Huang Di humbly replied, "Everything you have explained to me has been logical and of the deepest meaning. Although I cannot directly see the areas you have discussed, and I do not totally hear the numbers of which you speak, I am already much enlightened."

Qi Bo said, "This is what is meant by the saying, 'The sage easily comprehends, the good horse responds well to subtle commands.' "

Huang Di answered, "I am not the sage who comprehends easily. What I am trying to accomplish in asking these questions is to have you remove my cloudiness and inspire my development. Even this does not address the essence of the most important principles. But I hope you can, in as detailed a fashion as possible, explain the locations of the acupuncture points. This way, I will obtain an overview and also record and preserve the information in the *Golden Chamber*. I promise not to divulge the information to anybody other than the most appropriate ones."

Qi Bo bowed again. "I shall begin. When pain occurs in the back and radiates to the chest, or when pain occurs in the chest and radiates to the back, treatment involves acupuncturing tiantu (REN22) and zhongshu (DU7). Also use zhongwan (REN12), and guanyuan (REN4). Channels that traverse the back and chest are related to yin and yang. In the case of chest pain and associated back pain, causing shortness of breath, orthopnea, dyspnea, rapid breathing, or unilateral pain with fullness of the channels, the cause is in channels that traverse the rib area and connect the heart and diaphragm; go to the shoulder and tiantu (REN22), and diagonally move downward through the shoulder blades, around the level of the tenth thoracic vertebra.

"There are fifty acupuncture points bilaterally for the zang organs. There are seventy-two points bilaterally for the fu organs. There are fifty-nine points that deal with febrile disease. There are fifty-seven points that deal with water imbalance.* There are five rows of points on the scalp, with five points in each row; all together they equal twenty-five points. There are six back shu points corresponding to the five zang organs on the back; twelve of these in total bilaterally. There are two points along both sides of dazhui (DU14) called dashu (B11). On the sides of the eyes are two points, tongziliao (G1), and in front of the ears are fu bai (G10), also two points bilaterally. On both hips there are huantiao (G30), two points. There are the two dubi (ST35) points on the knee. There are two tinggong (SI19) points in front of the ear. There are the two zanzhu (B2) points of the eyebrow. On the scalp, there are the two wangu (G12) points. There is the fengfu (DU16) point under the external occipital protuberance. There are the two zhengu (G11) points in the back of the head. There are two shangguan (G3) points near the temple. There are two daying (ST5) points as well as two xiaquan (ST7) points in the jaws. There are two tianzhu (B10) points in the back of the neck. There are two shanglian (LI9) points and two xialian (LI8) points in the forearms. There are two jiache (ST6) in the face. There is the one tiantu (REN22) point below the throat. There are the two tianfu (LU3) points in the upper arms. There are the two tianyou (SJ16) points as well as two futu (LI18) points and two tianchuang (SI16) in the neck. There are two jianjing (G21) points in the shoulders. There is the one guanyuan (REN4) point in the abdomen. There are the two weiyang (B39) points behind the knees. There are the two jianzhen (SI9) points behind the shoulder joint. There is one yamean (DU15) point in the occiput. And in the belly button, there is the shenjue (REN8) point. There are twelve shu points of the chest. They are bulang (K22), shenfeng (K23), lingxu (K24), shencang (K25), yuzhong (K26), and shufu (K27) bilaterally on the chest. There are two shu points of the back and they are the geshu (B17) points

---

*The 50 points for the five zang organs include symmetrically, on each side of the body, five element points for each of the five zang organs. The 72 points for the fu organs include symmetrically, on each side of the body, five element points and yuan/source points for each of the six fu organs. The 59 points for febrile disease and the 57 points for water imbalance are both discussed in depth in chapter 61.

in the midback. There are twelve shu points of the pectoral chest area. There are two yangfu (G38) points in the calf area. There are two jiei (ST41) points in the foot. There are the two each of zhaohai (K6) points, which correspond to the yin qiao channel and shenmai (B62) points, which correspond to the yang qiao channel. There are two yangguan (G33) points that treat cold-induced conditions, which are located near the knees. There are two wuli (LI13) points, which are located five cun below tianfu (LU3), that are contraindicated for acupuncture. The above 365 acupuncture points are commonly used in treatment."

Huang Di said, "I finally grasp the location, application, and principles of the acupuncture points. But I would like to hear you discuss the luo or collaterals. Are the collaterals involved with the 365-day correspondence?"

Qi Bo replied, "The luo collaterals connect with the 365 points and correspond to the 365 days of the year. The function of the collaterals is to dispel the pathogen from the channels, and to promote the flow of the ying/nutritive and wei/defensive qi. When a pathogen attacks the body, causing the ying and the wei to stagnate, the wei qi disperses outward while the ying overflows inwardly. This causes fever and deficiency. Thus, one should sedate with acupuncture to promote flow within the collaterals. Wherever there is a change in skin color one should quickly sedate; do not worry whether this is a precise location for an acupuncture point."

Huang Di said, "Thank you for the clarification. Would you please discuss the areas you call xi and gu?"

Qi Bo answered, "Xi and gu areas, or small and large clefts, are where the bundles of muscles meet; at this meeting place there is a depression or indentation. These places of indentation or points collect the qi and act as canals in providing a conduit for the flow of qi to take place. If the pathogens allowed to linger in xi and gu, it will lead to stagnation of the qi and cause the channels and collaterals to heat up. This damages the muscles. If the ying and wei cannot get through, boils and abscesses result. Internally, the marrow can become depleted. Externally, ulcerations of the foot can result. If the pathogen lingers in the joints, degeneration occurs, with a poor prognosis. If a cold pathogen lingers, the ying and wei cannot properly flow. The tendomuscular meridians will then shrivel and one's limbs will become stiff. Internally, this causes bi of the bones. This is all due to severe cold factors lingering in the xi points. We consider this a deficient condition. The xi and gu points are also connected to the 365 points and correspond to one year. If the condition is fairly mild, creating mild stagnation where the pathogen is on the surface or traveling in the collaterals, one can easily treat with acupuncture. One would acupuncture the collaterals."

Huang Di bowed with respect and expressed his gratitude to Qi Bo. "Today you have inspired my further development and removed my questions and cloudiness. I shall record this wisdom carefully and preserve it in the *Golden Chamber*. I will not show it to anyone without due consideration."

Qi Bo concluded, "The various collaterals that connect throughout the body act as connectors that can be utilized to drain off the pathogen or to supply qi to combat illness. They consist of fourteen main collaterals with numerous tiny collaterals crisscrossing the body connecting the main channels with one another. However, when the deep level of the bones are attacked by a pathogen, the collaterals are insufficient and one must plunge the five main channels bilaterally that correspond to the five zang organs."

CHAPTER 59

PATHWAYS OF THE CHANNELS

Q I Bo said, "The foot taiyang/bladder channel traverses seventy-eight points bilaterally in all. It starts with a point on both eyebrows and travels up the forehead to connect with the du/governing channel. All together, its qi permeates five vertical pathways of five points each on the scalp, with the du channel at the midline with two rows on each side and three cun between the middle row and the outer row. Descending along the posterior aspect of the neck, crossing tianzhu (B10) and fengchi (G20) and proceeding downward parallel and about one and a half cun bilateral to the spine. From the first thoracic vertebra to the last vertebra of the sacrum there are a total of twenty-one vertebrae; there is a point corresponding to about fifteen of them. This part includes six shu points on each side that correspond to the zang organs. Finally the journey traverses down the leg; between weizhong (B40) in the back of the knee to the little toe there are six points on each leg.

"The foot shaoyang/gallbladder channel crosses a total of sixty-two points on both sides of the body. It begins at a point near the outer canthus; from the eyes to the scalp it counts five points on each side. Around the ear it crosses six points and connects with quepen (ST12) at the clavicle. Traveling to the side of the trunk, it moves through each point between every rib until the last rib, then moves to the hip, where it also has a point. The last section of the journey leads down the leg to the fourth toe; it counts six points on each leg.

"The foot yangming/stomach channel spans sixty-eight points on the body. From its origin on both sides of the nose it circles the face and forehead, connecting five points; it then runs down the neck and into the quepen (ST12) point at the clavicle. Traveling down the trunk, it passes through the nipple, crossing every point between the ribs until the umbilicus, where it connects with three points on each side about three cun from the midline. About two cun below the umbilicus it touches three more points before it emerges at the inguinal groove at qichong (ST30). Negotiating its way down the thigh, it crosses biquan (ST31) and futu (ST32) to the below the knee, where between zhusanli (ST36) and the middle toe it traverses eight points on each leg.

"The hand taiyang/small intestine channel crosses thirty-six points. Starting from the tip of the little finger, it travels up the arm, passing the elbow to the shoulder joint. Along the way it crosses seven points as it winds around the scapula, touching one point, and up the neck to tianchuang (SI16). It then travels to the cheek crossing from points and up to the side of the nose, connects with jingming (B1) at the inner canthus and tongziliao (G1) at the outer canthus of the eyes before it enters the ear on both sides.

"The hand yangming/large intestine channel traverses twenty-two points along its pathway. Starting at the index finger, it travels up the arm to the shoulder, passing six points in the process. From jianyu (LI15) at the shoulder it connects with a point in the clavicle and then turns upward through the face at daying (ST5) and two other points, and finally ends at the sides of the nose.

"The hand shaoyang/sanjiao channel crosses a total of thirty-two points. The qi flows from the fourth finger up the arm to the shoulder, crossing six points. Below the jianzhen (SI9) point of the shoulder it connects with three more points. Moving up the channel, it traverses around the ear and then the cheek and finally below the eye, crossing five points.

"The du/governing channel spans twenty-eight points on the body. Emerging from the tailbone, it travels up the spine until dazhui (DU14) at the seventh cervicle vertebra, crossing a total of fifteen points. Further up the neck, passing two points, it moves up the scalp to the top of the head and down the front of the face. Within the hairline it touches eight points. On the face it connects with three points.

"The ren/conception channel crosses twenty-eight points along its pathway. From the huiyin (REN1) at the perineum the channel moves up the midline of the body, passing six points between the pubic bone and the umbilicus. Further up to the chest it passes though four points between shangwan (REN13) and the umbilicus, and two points between jiwei (REN15) and shangwan (REN13). On the sternum it crosses six points, and in the throat it connects with two more points. Continuing its way into the face, it connects with a point below the lower lip and crosses another in the gum, finally ending at a point below the eyes.

"The chong/vitality channel traverses a total of twenty-two points. Measure half of a cun bilateral to the midline at the xiphoid process, and you will find the pathway moving down to the pubic bone. There is a point located at every cun spanning this distance.

"The foot shaoyin/kidney channel connects with two points on the underside of the tongue. The foot jueyin/liver channel possesses a point near the genitals called jimai (LV12). The hand shaoyin/heart channel has a xi/cleft point on both arms called yinxi (H6). The yinqiao/yin heel channel has a connecting point near the ankle called jiaoxin (K8) where as the yang-qiao/yang heel channel has a point on the outer ankle called fuyang (B59). Finally, the junction of dark and light skin in the hands and feet are also where the qi of all channels traverse."

Qi Bo concluded, "In summary, there are a total of 365 points that were just described."

CHAPTER 60

—

ACUPOINTS ALONG
SKELETAL INDENTATIONS

—

HUANG DI said, "I have heard that wind is the root of all illness. When using acupuncture to treat this, what kind of methods can one employ?"

Qi Bo replied, "When the wind pathogen attacks, it causes chills, sweating, headaches, heaviness, and aversion to wind. One must harmonize the yin and yang by acupuncturing fengfu (DU16), located above the first cervicle vertebra and below the external occipital protuberance. If the anti-pathogenic qi is weak, one should use the tonification method. If the pathogen is of an excess nature, one should sedate. After a more severe exposure to wind, one will manifest severe neck pain and stiffness. Acupuncture fengfu (DU16) again. If the patient is exposed to a 'big wind' and experiences sweating, the physician should moxa yixi (B45), which is located at the level of the sixth thoracic vertebra, three cun laterally. Palpate the point to elicit an 'yixi' expression (a painful exclamation) from the patient.

"With patients who are extremely averse to wind or drafts, one should acupuncture zanzhu (B2). For severe neck pain, one should moxa in the shoulder area at jianjing (G21). If the pain is like that of a fracture, moxa jizhong (DU6). To locate this point, ask the patient to bend the elbow while allowing the arm to hang down on the side. The point is on the spine at the level of the tip of the elbow joint.

"With pain that begins at the end of the ribs and travels to the lower abdomen, causing distension, one should acupuncture the yixi (B45) point. For low back pain with inability to rotate, severe muscle spasms, and pain that radiates to the scrotum, one should acupuncture the baliao points in the sacral foramen.

"With conditions of scrofula that include chills and fever, one should needle yangguan (G33) below the knee. When locating this point, have the patient bend forward as if bowing. The point is located superolateral to the knee. Incidently, when seeking points on the sole, have the patient kneel as if doing a salutation.

"Among the eight extraordinary channels, the ren/conception, du/ governing and chong/vitality are of the greatest importance. The ren/conception channel has its origin at huiyin (REN1). It travels from the perineum, up the abdomen, through guanyuan (REN4), and up to the throat. It continues to the eyes.

"The chong/vitality channel originates in qichong (ST30) in the groin. This is connected with the foot shaoyin/kidney channel. It moves upward with the kidney channel to the chest, where it disperses.

"In men, when the ren/conception channel is disordered, seven different types of hernia may develop; in women we will see leukorrhea and tumors. In disorders of the chong/vitality channel, the qi will rebel upward, causing acute abdominal pain and contracture.

"When the du/governing channel is disordered, the spine can become very stiff. The du/governing channel begins in the lower abdomen; in women, it begins in the urinary opening. A branch goes through the genitals and converges at huiyin (REN1). It then travels around the anal area and branches again through the thigh, where it connects with the foot shaoyin/ kidney channel. It combines with the luo/collateral of foot taiyang and foot shaoyin to converge in the buttocks. It travels upward from there, penetrating the spine and finally connecting with the kidneys. From here it combines with the foot taiyang channel, traveling to the eye area and forehead, crossing the vertex. It sends collaterals directly into the brain. It emerges from the head, descending to the anterior shoulder, goes back to the spine, and travels to the low back. It again enters the luo/collateral and connects with the kidneys. In males, the du/governing channel travels down from the kidneys through the root of the penis, converging at huiyin (REN1). The channel crosses the umbilicus, goes up through the heart into the throat and around the mouth, stopping below the eyes.

"In disorders of the du/governing channel, the qi may rush upward from the low abdomen into the heart or stomach, causing pain or subsequent obstruction of urine and bowels. This is called chong shan, or hiatal hernia. In women it causes infertility, difficulty urinating, hemorrhoids, or bedwetting. In general, the du/governing channel disorders call for acupuncturing the du/governing channel itself. In mild cases, acupuncture the qugu (REN2) point. In severe cases, acupuncture yinjiao (REN7).

If a patient has rebellious qi with rapid, hoarse breathing, acupuncture tiantu (REN22). If the rebellious qi emerges at the throat, acupuncture daying (ST5) point. When the knees can extend but cannot flex properly, one should acupuncture the biguan (ST31) point in the thigh. When one has knee pain sitting down, use the huantiao (G30) point. When the patient feels heat in the knee joint while standing, acupuncture the yangguan (G33) point by the knee. Knee pain radiating to the big toe calls for needling the weizhong (B40) point. When the patient is sitting and the knee feels as if something is inside, acupuncture the joint itself. When the knee has pain and cannot be extended, acupuncture the back points on the foot taiyang/bladder channel. If the pain is so severe that the tibia feels broken, acupuncture zhusanli (ST36). You may also use ying/spring points on the foot taiyang/bladder channel, tonggu (B66) and on the foot shaoyin/kidney channel, rangu (K2). When there is pain in the fibula and one cannot stand for long, acupuncture the guangming (G37) point.

"There are fifty-seven points that treat water disease. Above the buttocks are five rows with five points each. Above futu (ST32) in the abdomen there are two rows of five points each. To the left and right there is one row with five points. Above the medial ankle is one row with six points.

"There are many indentations or foramens in the various bones of the body that contain acupoints.

"When using moxibustion for wind cold conditions, begin with dazhui (DU14). The age of the patient determines how many moxa cones are used. Then moxa the coccyx. Observe the back for indentations and moxa those. In the rib area, one can moxa the jingmen (G25) points. On the outside of the upper ankle, one can moxa the xuanzhong (G39) point. On the toes there are the xiaxi (G43) points for moxibustion. There are also the chengshan (B57) point in the calf area and the kunlun (B60) point on the foot taiyang/bladder channel. The tender spots above the clavicle can also be treated this way. One can moxa the tiantu (REN22), yangchi (SJ4), guanyuan (REN4), zhusanli (ST36), chongyang (ST42), and baihai (DU20) points. To treat a dogbite, moxa with three cones at the site of the bite. These twenty-nine points are useful for moxibustion treatments. When fever and chills are caused by food poisoning or stomach flu that do not respond to moxibustion treatment, the illness is due to an excess of heat pathogen. In this case acupuncture the shu/stream points on the overheated channel at frequent intervals in order to disperse the pathogen and rectify the imbalance."

CHAPTER 61

—

ACUPUNCTURE TREATMENT IN WATER AND FEBRILE DISEASES

——

HUANG DI asked, "Why does the shaoyin correspond to the kidneys, and why do the kidneys dominate water metabolism?"

Qi Bo answered, "The kidneys are located at the lowest point of the trunk; they are yin within yin. It is the extreme yin of all the organs. Extreme yin corresponds to water, which is of yin quality. The lung also is involved in water metabolism of the upper trunk; it is called hand taiyin whereas the kidney is known as foot shaoyin. Shaoyin is most dominant in the winter. Water and edema conditions have their root in the kidney and their manifestations in the lung. Both organs are capable of accumulating water and manifesting disease."

Huang Di asked, "Why does the kidney retain water and cause illness?"

Qi Bo replied, "The kidney is the outer door to the stomach. When the door does not open and close properly, water is retained and causes illness. The water then proceeds into the tissues and under the skin to cause swelling."

Huang Di said, "According to this, all water and water-related swelling conditions have their root in the kidney."

Qi Bo answered, "The kidney organs are yin organs. Anything that has to do with steaming upward of the earth qi has to do with the kidneys. The kidneys process fluid from the body by applying qi and yang, thereby refining the fluid into a mist that lubricates the body. We consider this a very extreme yin quality.

"Let us take an example of someone who is physically strained and becomes exhausted, which depletes the kidneys and results in dehydration from sweating. As the person sweats there is an attack of wind, which causes the pores to suddenly close. The sweat is now trapped; it can neither return to the zang fu nor be expelled. It accumulates and causes swelling. The root of this is in the kidneys. It is called feng shui, or wind-water syndrome."

Huang Di said, "There are fifty-seven points one can use to treat water disease. What are those points controlled by?"

Qi Bo answered, "The kidneys, of course. This is where the yin qi converges. It is also where water is transported. Along the sacral area there are five vertical rows of points, each with five points. They are changqiang (DU1), yaoshu (DU2), mingmen (DU4), xuanshu (DU5), and juzhong (DU6) on the du/governing channel; dachangshu (B25), xiaochangshu (B27), pangguanshu (B28), zhonglushu (B29), baihuanshu (B 30), weicang (B50), huangmen (B51), zhishi (B52), baohuang (B53), and zhibian (B54) on the bladder channel. These are points controlled by the kidneys. When water is so severe that it floods the lower half of the body, or when the abdomen retains water, we find orthopnea and dyspnea in the upper body. This is biao ben tong bing, the cause and the manifestation. That is, the kidney is the cause, while the lung is the manifestation.

"Above the thighs in the abdomen there are two rows of five points on each side. They are henggu (K11), dahe (K12), qixue (K13), siman (K14), and zhongzhu (K15); wailing (ST26), daju (ST27), shuidao (ST28), guilai (ST29), and qichong (ST30). This is the pathway transversed by the kidney qi, therefore referred to as the thoroughfare of the kidneys. The liver, kidney, and spleen channels converge on the inside of the leg. The kidney channel counts six points on each leg, collectively called taichong, or the great thoroughfare. They consist of dazhong (K4), zhaohai (K6), fuliu (K7), jiaoxin (K8), zhubin (K9), and yingu (K10). All fifty-seven points are where the pathogenic water may linger and hence are used to disperse the stagnation of water pathogens."

Huang Di said, "During the spring, one should acupuncture between the luo collaterals and the flesh. Why is this?"

Qi Bo replied, "The spring corresponds to wood and liver, which have to do with growth and vitality. The liver qi is one of quick temper and impatience. It moves suddenly, like the wind. The main channels generally travel deeply. When the wind pathogen begins, it usually attacks the superficial levels and has not penetrated into the main channels. Thus we need only to insert needles shallowly to reach between the luo collaterals and the flesh level."

Huang Di asked, "What about acupuncturing during the summer?

Then one generally inserts superficially in the major channels. Why is this?"

Qi Bo replied, "The summer corresponds to heart and fire. It is a period of robust growth. Within the channels the qi is relatively weak. In fact, the channels are relatively narrow at this time. But the yang qi and heat are very strong. This heat comes from the outside and burns its way into the channels. In this case, one should locate the channel in which there is excess. Then needle points on the major channel through the skin and the pathogen will simply vanish. The pathogen is at a superficial level and is easily defeated."

Huang Di said, "When one acupunctures in the autumn, one should find the shu/stream points on the major channels. Why is this?"

Qi Bo replied, "The autumn corresponds to metal and the lung. This is a time of suppressive, harsh energy and climate. Metal is excess and the fire has weakened. The yang qi circulates in the he/sea points. Yin qi is beginning to rise and the damp pathogen can invade the body. However, the pathogen is still not strong enough to penetrate deeply. Thus, locate the shu/stream points to arrest and dispel the yin pathogen. Treat the he/sea points for yang pathogens."

Huang Di said, "In the winter, we use the jing/well and rong/spring points. Why is this?"

Qi Bo answered, "The winter corresponds to water and the kidney. It is the start of storing and hibernating. Yang qi has weakened, yin qi is very strong. Yang qi sinks deep within. Thus we need to use jing/well points to manage the yin, to drain off yin pathogen. We then use rong/spring points to strengthen the counteracting yang qi, thus achieving balance. There is a saying: 'In winter find the jing/well and rong/spring points to balance yin and yang—thus in spring one can prevent nosebleeds from yang rising.' "

Huang Di said, "I am grateful for your explanation of the treatment methods of febrile disease, using fifty-nine points. I have a general grasp of them. But can you tell me the location of the points, and enlighten me as to their functions?"

Qi Bo answered, "On the scalp there are five vertical rows of five points each. They can treat any kind of heat pathogen that rises to the head. They are on the du/governing channel, houding (DU19), baihui (DU20), qianding (DU21), xinhui (DU22), and shangxing (DU23); and on the bladder channel, wuchu (B5), chengguang (B6), tongtian (B7), luoque (B8), yuzhen

(B9); and on the gallbladder channel, lingqi (G15), muchuang (G16), zhen-gying (G17), chengling (G18), and naokong (G19). There are eight points that can eliminate heat in the chest. They are dashu (B11), yingshu, quepen (ST12), and beishu. There are eight points that can eliminate heat in the stomach. They are qichong (ST 30), zhusanli (ST36), shanglian (LI9), and xialian (LI8). There are eight points that can eliminate heat in the four extremities. They are yunmen (LU2), jianyu (LI15), weizhong (B40), and naokong (G19). There are five points that eliminate heat in the organs that are on the back that correspond to each of the five zang organs. They are pohu (B42), shentang (B44), hunmen (B47), yishe (B49), and zhishi (B52). These sum up the fifty-nine points can be used in treating febrile disease."

Huang Di said, "How does an attack of a cold pathogen transform into febrile disease?"

Qi Bo replied simply, "The extreme of cold will stagnate and turn into heat."

CHAPTER 62

—

REGULATION OF THE CHANNELS

—

Huang Di said, "I have heard that in applying techniques of acupuncture, one should use sedation techniques for excess conditions and tonification techniques for deficiency conditions. What is meant by excess and deficiency?"

Qi Bo replied, "There are five types of excess and five types of deficiency. Which are you inquiring about?"

Huang Di said, "I would like to learn about them all."

Qi Bo said, "Shen, or spirit, can be excess or deficient. Qi can be excess or deficient. Blood can be excess or deficient. The form can be excess or deficient. The zhi, or will, can also be excess or deficient. These constitute ten types."

Huang Di said, "In the human being there are jing/essence, qi, jin ye or body fluids, four extremities, nine orifices, five zang organs, sixteen channels,* and three hundred and sixty-five joints. All are capable of becoming disordered and diseased. In each disorder there are distinctions of deficiency and excess. Now, my teacher, you have mentioned only five types of deficiency and excess. Can you please expound upon this?"

Qi Bo replied, "The five types of excess and deficiency are borne from the five zang organs. For example, the heart houses the shen or spirit; the lungs house the qi; the liver accommodates the blood; the spleen houses the form and flesh; and the kidneys house the zhi, or will. They must all function together as the zhi and the shen are functioning in concert psychically, connecting with the bones and marrow within and forming the shape of the body without. This creates an entire functional being and is the makeup of the human body. Within the five zang, communication occurs via pathways or channels, which transport the qi and blood. When the qi

_____

*Sixteen Channels include the twelve major channels, adding du/governing, ren/conception, dai/belt, and chong/vitality channels.

and blood are not regulated, illness occurs. Diagnosis and treatment are thus dependent on the channels and pathways."

Huang Di asked, "Will you please tell me about conditions where the shen is excess or deficient?"

Qi Bo answered, "When the shen is excessive, one laughs hysterically. When the shen is deficient, one is sad or crying. This occurs only when a pathogen disrupts the qi and blood, causing a disturbance in the zang. Before the pathogen disrupts the qi and blood, however, one experiences an eerie chill. This is still a mild pathologic condition of the shen."

Huang Di asked, "How do you utilize tonification and sedation techniques to treat this?"

Qi Bo replied, "If the shen is excess, bleed the tiny luo collaterals, but shallowly, without much of an opening, and not in the major channels. This will return the shen to a calm state. When the shen is deficient, locate the deficient luo that is associated with the shen. Begin by performing massage, then administer acupuncture to promote qi and blood flow. Do not allow either to escape from the channels. In this way, the shen will return to tranquillity."

Huang Di asked, "When treating mild pathogens with acupuncture, what needs to be done?

Qi Bo answered, "Massage, or tuina, followed by acupuncture is effective, as long as one takes care not to cause large openings from the needles. Then direct the qi to move to the area of deficiency and thus restore the shen."

Huang Di replied, "Thank you, now I understand. Can you please discuss the excesses and deficiencies of the qi?"

Qi Bo answered, "When the qi is excess, one has dyspnea and cough; the qi rebels upward. When the qi is deficient, there is shortness of breath. Before the disruption of the qi and blood by the pathogens, the condition is one of slight lung qi deficiency."

Huang Di asked, "And how do you apply the techniques of tonification and sedation?"

Qi Bo answered, "When the qi is excess, sedate the channels without causing injury. Do not allow blood to escape. In deficiency, tonify the channels. Do not allow qi to escape."

Huang Di asked, "How do you acupuncture in a mild condition?"

Qi Bo replied, "Massage is a good modality. Also take out needles and show them to the patient. Verbalize the acupuncture procedure so that the patient will be slightly apprehensive, thus causing the qi to withdraw inward. Then insert the needle to the appropriate depth and dispel the pathogen. When the pores open and sweat occurs, withdraw the needle and the body will naturally recover."

Huang Di asked, "Will you please tell me about excess and deficient conditions of the blood?"

Qi Bo answered, "When the blood is excess, one gets angry. When the blood is deficient, one is fearful. Before the qi and blood are disrupted, an excess condition will manifest in the tiny luo collaterals. As it becomes more excessive, it flows into the major channels. This causes stagnation of blood in the channels."

Huang Di asked, "Can you explain techniques of tonification and sedation in relation to this?"

Qi Bo replied, "When the blood is excess, sedate the channel that is filled. Perform minor bloodletting. In deficiency, locate the proper channel and perform acupuncture on it. Leave the needles in as you examine the patient's pulses. If the pulse is flooding and large, immediately withdraw the needle. Do not allow bleeding."

Huang Di asked, "What is the procedure when the blood is stagnant in the channels?"

Qi Bo answered, "Locate that channel; perform acupuncture and bloodletting. This allows the blood to escape the channel and disperse the stagnation."

Huang Di said, "Thank you, now I understand. Can you please discuss excess and deficiency of the form and flesh?"

Qi Bo replied, "When the form is excess, the abdomen is distended and large and there is difficult urination. When the form is deficient, the extremities are difficult to mobilize. Before the pathogen disrupts the qi, blood, and the five zang, one may find that the muscles will twitch. This is called minor wind."

Huang Di said, "Please tell me how to apply tonification and sedation techniques."

Qi Bo answered, "In excess conditions of the flesh, sedate the foot yangming or stomach channel. In deficiency, tonify the same."

Huang Di inquired, "How do you approach the minor wind condition?"

Qi Bo replied, "Acupuncture within the flesh to disperse the pathogen; do not needle all the way to the channel or injure the luo. Thus, the wei or defensive qi can slowly recover while the pathogenic qi will gradually vanish."

Huang Di asked, "Will you please discuss excess and deficiency of zhi/will?"

Qi Bo answered, "When the zhi/will is excess, there is abdominal distension and diarrhea of undigested food. When the zhi/will is deficient there is extreme cold in the hands and feet. Before the pathogenic qi disrupts the body's qi, blood, and zang organs, one finds crepitation within the joints as if the bones are rattling."

Huang Di inquired, "How do you tonify and sedate in this case?"

Qi Bo answered, "In an excess of zhi/will, acupuncture and perform bloodletting at the rangu (K2) point. In deficiency, tonify at the fuliu (K7) point. In mild cases where there is crepitation, acupuncture the affected joint and thus do not allow the pathogen to progress to the main channels. In this way the pathogen will be successfully repelled."

Huang Di said, "Thank you for expounding on these conditions of excess and deficiency. Now can you tell me how these come about?"

Qi Bo answered, "The causes of excess and deficiency have to do with the interaction of the pathogen and the body's qi, blood, yin, and yang. When the yin and yang become imbalanced, the wei qi becomes chaotic, and the blood becomes rebellious in the channels. The blood and qi become nonconforming and stray from their normal paths. This leads to excess and deficiency. For example, when the blood is excess in the yin level while the qi is excess in the yang level, the patient will manifest mania and violence. If the blood is excess in the yang and the qi is excess in the yin, the patient will manifest febrile disease. If the blood is excess at the top while the qi is excess at the bottom, the patient will be irritable, restless, and easily angered, and will feel a sensation of fullness in the chest. If the blood is excess in the lower while the qi is excess in the upper, the patient will lose his mind and become forgetful."

Huang Di asked, "When the blood is excess in the yin level while the qi is excess in the yang level, and the qi and blood diverge from their normal paths, how does one truly determine what is excess and what is deficient?"

Qi Bo answered, "The qi and blood prefer an environment of warmth and dislike cold. Cold causes both to stagnate, while warmth aids their flow. In places where the qi is excess, the blood becomes diminished. Where the blood is excess, the qi is insufficient."

Huang Di said, "Within the human body we are discussing qi and blood. As you have said, my teacher, when qi and blood are excess, one can still manifest deficient conditions. Does this mean that the excess is not real?"

Qi Bo answered, "Excess means that there is extra, that is all. Deficient means that there is not enough. Where the qi is excessive, the blood can become displaced and deficient. Where the blood is excess, the qi can become displaced and deficient. Because the qi and blood have lost their quantitative harmony, the result is deficiency of one aspect relative to the other. In the tiny luo and main luo collaterals, there exist blood and qi that are being transported to the major channels. If both qi and blood are excessive here, it can cause crowding in the channels and therefore it is an excess condition. If the blood and qi are both excess in the channels, they can become rebellious. This is called da jui, major syncope, where one loses consciousness suddenly. If the physician can quickly reverse the rebellious flow of the qi and blood, resuscitation is possible. If reversal cannot be achieved, however, the consequence is death."

Huang Di asked, "Where does excess come from and what is the significance of deficiency? Can you please explain what brings these conditions on?"

Qi Bo answered, "The yin and yang channels possess shu or what is called stream points, where transportation and convergence of qi and blood occur. Blood and qi of a yang channel will transport to the yin channels. The yin channels then fill and nourish the body. When yin and yang are balanced, the body becomes robust. The nine locations of the body's pulses will also be in concert. This occurs in a normal, healthy person. A pathogen may attack the body, causing imbalance and bringing on either a condition of a yin nature that affects the zang internally, or a yang disease on the body's surface. A yin condition typically arises from improper diet, a lack of regularity in lifestyle, excess sex, or lack of harmonious emotions. A yang condition is typically brought on by exposure to rain, wind, cold, or summer heat."

Huang Di said, "How do wind and rain injure people?"

Qi Bo answered, "The wind and rain first attack the skin. Then they move to the smaller luo, the regular luo, and finally to the major channels. When the pathogen arrives in the major channels, it disrupts qi and blood flow, causing stagnation. This is why we find a strong and large pulse, an excess condition. In excess conditions, the surface of the body feels tight, stiff, hard, and full, and there is a dislike of being touched because of pain."

Huang Di asked, "Can you tell me how cold and damp injure people?"

Qi Bo replied, "These cause the skin's surface to lose its elasticity. The muscles become tight and hard, which in turn stagnates the flow of ying or nutritive qi and blood. This causes the wei or defensive qi to weaken, a deficient condition. Deficiency manifests with a flaccid skin full of wrinkles; touching the skin warms and fortifies the qi and is comforting to the patient."

Huang Di asked, "Will you please explain the excess condition that occurs in the yin level or interior of the body?"

Qi Bo answered, "When the emotions are not regulated and one indulges in them, a situation is created where the yin qi moves abnormally upward, leaving the lower body deficient. When the lower body is deficient in yin, the yang qi moves in and fills the void, causing an excess state."

Huang Di asked, "What happens in a deficiency state of yin?"

Qi Bo replied, "Overindulgence in excitement and joy causes the qi to scatter. Indulgence in sadness exhausts the qi. When the qi is exhausted, the channels become empty. If one simultaneously eats cold and raw foods, coldness will permeate the interior. In this circumstance the blood flow will become slow and choppy along with exhaustion of the qi. This is known as deficiency."

Huang Di said, "In ancient medical treatises, yang deficiency is mentioned as causing coldness in the exterior. Yin deficiency causes heat to rise in the interior. When yang is excess, heat manifests on the exterior. Yin excess causes coldness on the interior. Can you please tell me the mechanisms behind this?"

Qi Bo answered, "All the body's yang comes from the upper jiao or cavity. The function of this yang is to warm the skin and regulate the pores. If the cold pathogen attacks from the exterior, the qi of the upper jiao becomes stagnant. Cold accumulates in the exterior and causes chills."

Huang Di asked, "Can you explain yin deficiency causing heat?"

Qi Bo replied, "Overtiring oneself depletes the yin. The spleen and stomach are then inefficient in processing nutrients. The upper jiao cannot disperse the extracted nutrients, nor can the middle jiao assimilate them.

The stomach qi stagnates, leading to heat production. This heat then rises and permeates the chest. The result is internal heat."

Huang Di asked, "Will you please explain yang excess causing fever in the outer body?"

Qi Bo answered, "Because the upper jiao is unable to disperse, the pores cannot be regulated. Sweat is retained and the wei qi cannot perform its function. Heat then collects under the skin, resulting in fever."

Huang Di said, "Please tell me about yin excess causing internal cold."

Qi Bo said, "The disordered qi moves upward, bringing with it the cold that stagnates in the chest. When the yang qi cannot warm and dispel the cold, the blood stagnates. Next the entire channel system is disrupted; we then find a pulse that is big, excess, and choppy."

Huang Di asked, "When the yin and yang stagnate and are excess, and the blood and qi are not harmonized, an illness is certain to manifest. How then would one proceed with treatment?"

Qi Bo replied, "In treating such a condition, one should locate the channel and perform acupuncture reaching to the ying or nutritive level to treat the blood, and to the wei or defensive level to treat the qi. Take into account the various constitutions of a patient's body, as well as the particular season, in order to determine how much is appropriate."

Huang Di said, "At the point when the pathogen has contacted and disturbed the qi and blood, yin and yang have been imbalanced. How do you then apply your techniques?"

Qi Bo replied, "For sedation, have the patient inhale upon insertion of the needle. This causes the qi and the needle to enter the body simultaneously. This opens the door and allows the pathogen to exit. When withdrawing the needle, have the patient exhale so that the qi and the needle exit simultaneously. The body's jing/essence qi is thereby left uninjured, but the pathogen is dispelled. Do not block the opening made by the needle. Let the pathogen leave. You may have to move the needle in order to enlarge the exit point. This is considered intense sedation. When taking out the needle quickly, press with your left thumb at the point of exit to close the point after the pathogen is dispelled."

Huang Di asked, "Will you please tell me about tonification?"

Qi Bo replied, "Do not insert the needles right away. Concentrate your mind; then wait until the patient exhales before needling. Do not shake the needle; to contain the jing qi, be sure that there is no leakage around the needle. As soon as the de qi or qi arrives, withdraw the needles

as the patient inhales. Press on the opening. There is a definite limit to the
needle retention; as soon as the qi arrives, remove the needles. This prevents the qi in the surrounding areas from leaking. Also the qi may be
summoned from distant areas; thus, it is crucial not to lose it."

Huang Di said, "You mentioned ten types of excess and deficiency
caused within the five zang organs, but you have not made mention of the
twelve channels, which also can become imbalanced and manifest excesses
and deficiencies of their own. Will you discuss excess and deficiency disorders of the channels and how they relate to the five zang?"

Qi Bo replied, "The zang and fu viscera have internal and external
connections and correspondences with the channels. Each manifests excess
and deficient conditions that should be addressed according to their location. If the disease is in the channels, attend the blood. If the disease is in
the blood, adjust the luo. If the disease is in the qi, attend the wei. If the
disease is in the flesh, attend the flesh. If the disease is in the tendons,
address the tendons. If in the bones, treat the bones. In conditions where
there is bi or wind damp factors in the tendons, use the warm needle
technique where flame is applied to the needle after it is inserted. In diseased bones, use fire needle technique where the needle is hot and red
before it is inserted, or apply hot herbal compresses to the affected area. If
there is numbness, perform acupuncture to the yinqiao and yangqiao channels. If there is pain in the body but the nine pulses are normal, acupuncture
the luo. If the pain is on the left side, but there is pathology on the right
pulses, acupuncture the channels employing the opposite-side treatment
method. Apply treatment quickly. In every instance, examine the pulses of
the nine locations carefully before applying treatment. This ensures the
accuracy of your treatment and techniques."

CHAPTER 63

ACUPUNCTURING
THE SUPERFICIAL LUO

HUANG DI said, "I have heard of a technique that employs acupuncturing the superficial luo. Will you please tell me about this method and its indications?"

Qi Bo answered, "In general, when a pathogen invades the body, it first enters the skin level. If it lingers or is not expelled, it will travel into the micro luo. If still not expelled, it then travels to the regular luo channels. From here it proceeds into the main channels, connecting to the five zang organs, and finally to the intestines and stomach. At this stage, everything may be affected; the five zang will certainly suffer injury. This is the progression of the pathogen from the skin level into the five zang organs. One then needs to needle the normal acupuncture points.

"If the pathogen lingers in the micro luo and stagnates there, unusual diseases may occur. As the major luo are invaded, the pathogen will travel to the right if it originates from the left, and vice versa. It follows the pathways of the major luo into the extremities. If it does not invade the major channels, the pathogen may continue moving without a fixed location in the luo channels. If it is located on the right side, symptoms may appear on the left, and vice versa. When acupuncturing, utilize the procedure of treating the opposite side. The name for this method is miu ci, acupuncturing the superficial luo by opposite insertion."

Huang Di said, "I would like to hear you explain this miu ci method and treating disease on the opposite side. I am also curious about the differences between this and the treatment of the major channels."

Qi Bo answered, "When the pathogen attacks the channels and is abundant on the left side, the right side will be impacted. The reverse is also true. Acupuncture should be performed on the major channels. However, you must target the proper channel; treating only the luo channel is not sufficient. Symptoms of the luo disorders differ from those of the major channels."

Huang Di asked, "How exactly do you utilize miu ci?"

Qi Bo replied, "For example, if the pathogen attacks the luo of the foot shaoyin/gallbladder, the patient manifests heart pain, abdominal distension, and hypochondriac fullness. If there is no obvious stagnation, one can acupuncture the rangu (K2) point and perform bloodletting. Within thirty minutes the disease will likely be remedied. If not, however, use the technique of treating the opposite side. The illness will resolve within five days.

"When the pathogen enters the luo of the hand shaoyang/sanjiao, it can cause throat pain and constriction, contracture of the tongue, dry mouth, restlessness, irritability, and pain on the lateral portions of the arms. The patient cannot raise the hands above the head. Acupuncture the guanchong (SJ1) point on the fourth finger. If the patient is constitutionally strong, healing will be immediate. If the patient is older and weaker, healing will take longer. Certainly, one should apply the principle of needling the opposite side. If the condition is acute, healing will still occur within a few days.

"When the pathogen attacks the luo of the foot jueyin/liver, sudden painful hernia can result. In this case, acupuncture dadun (LIV1), on the big toe. In men the effect will be immediate; in women it will take slightly longer. Use the opposite point selection technique.

"If the pathogen attacks the luo of the foot taiyang/bladder, pain will result in the neck and shoulders. Needle the zhiyin (B67) point on the little toe and healing will occur. If this fails, needle jingmen (B63) three times on the opposite side. Results will occur within about thirty minutes.

"When the pathogen attacks the luo of the hand yangming/large intestine, chest fullness, dyspnea, fullness of the ribs, and feverish feeling in the chest will occur. Acupuncture the shangyang (LI1) point. Choose the opposite side. Results will occur within about thirty minutes.

"When the pathogen attacks the luo of the hand jueyin, pain in the wrists results, with lack of mobility. Acupuncture around the middle of the wrist. Find the painful point with your thumb, then insert the needle. Follow the lunar cycle when acupuncturing. Do this daily for fifteen days, from new moon to full moon, increasing the number of insertions by one each day. Then from full moon to the following new moon, decrease the number of insertions by one each day.

"When the pathogen attacks the yangqiao channel, eye pain will result. Acupuncture the shenmai (B62) point twice on the opposite side. Leave the needle in forty-five minutes. This will induce healing.

"If a patient comes to you after suffering a fall, which causes the blood to stagnate, there may be abdominal fullness and swelling, and obstruction of the bladder or rectum. Here one must immediately dispense herbs to open up the bladder and rectum. If the injury is on the top of the body, there will likely be injury to the jueyin channels. If the injury is to the lower portion, however, injury is to the shaoyin luo. Acupuncture on the inside of the ankle; bleed the capillary in front of rangu (K2). Also acupuncture chongyang (ST42). If there is no result, acupuncture dadun (LIV1), and perform bloodletting. Again, utilize the opposite side. If there is anxiety or fear and depression, repeat this procedure.

"If the pathogen enters the hand yangming luo, deafness or intermittent deafness can occur. Needle shangyang (LI1) to restore hearing. If there is no result, needle zhongchong (P9) to effect a cure. If there is total deafness and the luo qi has been depleted, do not use acupuncture. If the patient hears sounds like wind blowing, use these techniques with the opposing side method.

"In bi conditions where pain travels and is not fixed, one should apply acupuncture to the painful areas. Do this in accordance with the lunar cycle I mentioned earlier. Take into consideration the relative strength of the pathogen and the body in determining your approach and frequency. If one acupunctures more than the appropriate number of times, one can deplete the body's qi and cause the condition to worsen. If one acupunctures too infrequently, one will not achieve complete benefit. Again, employ the method of the opposite side and adhere to the lunar cycle.

"When a pathogen enters the luo of the foot yangming, it causes sneezing, nosebleeds, and coldness in the upper teeth. Acupuncture the lidui (ST45) point. Of course, utilize the principle of needling the opposite side.

"When a pathogen attacks the luo of the foot shaoyang/gallbladder, it causes discomfort in breathing, cough with spontaneous sweating, and rib or chest pain. One should acupuncture the fourth toe at zhuqiaoyin (G44). This will immediately relieve the breathing difficulty and stop sweating. For the cough, advise the patient regarding diet and proper dress. This will resolve within one day. However, if the patient does not heal, repeat the procedure.

"If the pathogen attacks the luo of the foot shaoyin, it can cause throat pain, difficulty swallowing, anger without apparent reason, and qi that rebels up to the cardiac orifice. One should acupuncture yongchuan (K1), three times on each side. This should produce immediate results. If not, however, repeat the procedure using the other side. If the throat swells so as to cause complete obstruction, one should acupuncture rangu (K2) and perform bloodletting.

"When a pathogen attacks the luo of the foot taiyin/spleen, it causes low back pain that radiates to the low abdomen and the ribs. The patient cannot sit upright and breathe. Acupuncture the points along the sacrum and in the sacral foramen, as well as the shu points. The frequency of needling should follow the lunar cycle. One can expect immediate results.

"When a pathogen attacks the luo of the foot taiyang, it causes sudden spasms of the back, and pain that radiates from the back to the ribs. Follow along the neck, down both sides of the spine, and acupuncture the painful spots three times.

"When the pathogen attacks the luo of the foot shaoyang, it causes pain in the hip and difficulty flexing the thigh. Employ very long and thin needles in treating huantiao (G30). If the cold pathogen is dominant, leave the needle in longer. Acupuncture frequency depends on the lunar cycle. One should achieve immediate results.

"When treating channel pathology, if the manifestation is not along the pathway of the major channels but rather along the luo, use the miu ci method. The reverse is also true: if the miu ci method is ineffective, the illness may have penetrated the major channels. With deafness, for example, when one uses the shangyang (LI1) point of hand yangming without result, we should try the tinggong (SI19) point in front of the ear. For a tooth cavity, if the same shangyang (LI1) point does not work, we should acupuncture the luo collaterals that travel to the teeth.

"When a pathogen attacks deeply at the zang organ level, we find radiating pain that may be intermittent. The physician can begin with a luo treatment of the miu ci variety, using the webs of the hands and feet. Choose the luo collaterals that have blood stagnation and perform bloodletting. Acupuncture every other day. If the first treatment does not succeed, healing will occur after five treatments.

"When the hand yangming channel is diseased and the pathogen travels up to the teeth, resulting in pain and coldness of the lips and teeth, observe the back of the hand to find congealed blood. Dispel this congealed blood by bloodletting, then acupuncture the lidui (ST45) and the shangyang (LI1) points to achieve immediate results.

"When the pathogen enters the luo of the hand shaoyin, foot shaoyin, hand taiyin, foot taiyin, or foot yangming channels, all of which meet in the ear, especially at the forehead above the left ear, the qi of these five luo may become depleted. This causes the entire body to be affected. A total loss of sensation and consciousness may occur, as if one is dead. This is called shi jue. Acupuncture yinbai (SP1); then yongchuan (K1); then lidui (ST45); then shaoshang (LU11); then zhongchong (P9); then shenmen (H7). If there is no effect, utilize hollow bamboo straws to blow into both the patient's ears. First, shave off a section of hair at the left side of the forehead. Burn this, make a powder, and mix this with rice wine. Force-feed this into the patient to aid in recovery.

"In general, when contemplating methods of acupuncture, one should determine the channel that is affected. Then determine whether it is excess or deficiency. Follow this with the appropriate treatment. If the blood in the channels is not functioning properly, acupuncture the malfunctioning channel. If there is pain that is not on the major channel pathways, utilize the luo treatment. Pay special attention to areas of stagnation and dispel the pathogen through bloodletting. Utilize point selection on the side opposite the symptoms. All these constitute miu ci method, or acupuncturing the superficial luo."

CHAPTER 64

—

ACUPUNCTURE
ACCORDING TO THE SEASONS

—

Huang Di said, "If the qi in the jueyin channel is excessive, a condition called yin bi, or extreme yin stagnation, can result. When there is a deficiency, a condition of re bi, or heat bi, can result. If there is a slippery pulse, a condition of shan or hernia, which occurs intermittently, can result. If there is a choppy pulse, we suspect a stagnation of qi in the lower abdomen.

"When the qi in the shaoyin channel is excessive, a patient may manifest bi in the skin level or a rash. When the qi is deficient, there will be bi in the lung. With a slippery pulse, there is hernia that is induced by external wind. This is known as lung wind hernia. A choppy pulse may mean accumulation conditions with hematuria.

"When the qi in the taiyin channel is excess, one might see bi in the flesh and coldness in the middle jiao. Deficiency in the taiyin channel would mean bi in the spleen. A slippery pulse indicates hernia or spleen wind. A choppy pulse indicates accumulation with fullness and distension of the epigastrium and abdomen.

"When the qi in the yangming channel is excessive, there is bi in the vessels, along with fever. When the qi is deficient, there will be bi of the chest and heart. A slippery pulse indicates hernia or heart wind. A choppy pulse indicates stagnation, anxiety, and a patient who is easily startled.

"When the qi is excess in the taiyang channel, the manifestation may be bi of the bones, causing heaviness throughout the body. When the qi is deficient, there will be bi of the kidneys. A slippery pulse indicates hernia or kidney wind. A choppy pulse indicates retention and disorders at the vertex of the head.

"When the qi in the shaoyang is excess, there will be bi of the tendons and fullness in the ribs. When the qi is deficient, there may be bi of the liver. A slippery pulse indicates hernia or liver wind. A choppy pulse indicates retention and spasm of the tendons and eye pain.

"In these conditions, the qi of the channels corresponds to the qi of the four seasons. In the spring, the wood/wind qi travels in the channels. In the summer, the heart/fire qi travels in the micro luos. In the late summer, the wet earth qi travels in the flesh. In the autumn, the dry metal qi travels in the skin. In the winter, the cold water qi travels in the bone marrow."

Huang Di said, "I would like to understand the underlying reasons for this phenomenon."

Qi Bo replied, "In the spring, the yang qi of the universe begins to grow. The yin qi of the earth begins to disperse. Coldness turns to warmth. Ice melts. Water flows into the streams and rivers. The qi in the human body flows in the channels. In the summer, the blood and qi overflow with abundance in the channels. They flow into the micro luo. The skin is nourished and strong. In the late summer, the qi and blood in the channels and luo are both abundant. The nourishment and lubrication of the muscles take place. By the autumn, as the earth takes energy back, the pores of the body begin to close, and the skin shrinks. By the winter the energy is of hibernating and storing. Similarly, the qi of the body turns inward to the deepest level, the bone marrow. From there, the qi flows to the five zang organs.

"Pathogenic qi also follows this movement throughout the four seasons. Its changes, however, are dynamic and unpredictable. In treatment, one should still follow the principles of the movement of the four seasons. This will enable one to completely eradicate pathogens from the body."

Huang Di asked, "In treatment, if one violates the principles of the qi flow of the four seasons, causing reckless movement of the qi and blood within the system, what would this bring on?"

Qi Bo answered, "In the spring the qi is in the channels. Thus, if one treated the luo instead of the channel, the qi and blood would disperse outward, leading to shortness of breath. If one punctured the muscle layer, the qi and blood flow would be disrupted, leading to asthma and dyspnea. If one treated the tendon and bone layer, the qi and blood would be retained in the interior, leading to distension of the abdomen.

"In the summer the qi should be flowing into the luo. If one treats the channels, the qi will become exhausted, leading to fatigue and sluggishness. If one treats the muscle layer, the qi and blood will be depleted, leading to fright. If one treats the tendon and bone layer, the qi and blood will rebel upward, causing anger.

"In the fall the qi is in the skin. If one treats the channels, the qi and blood will rebel upward, causing forgetfulness. If one treats the luo, the qi cannot circulate to the surface. This causes hypersomnia and laziness. If one treats the tendon and bone layer, the chaos of qi and blood leads to shivering and chills.

"In the winter the qi and blood are deep in the bone and marrow level. If one treats the channels, the qi and blood will cause a temporary deficit, leading to a decrease in vision. If one treats the luo, the qi will pour outward, causing bi of the five zang organs. If one treats the muscle layer, the yang qi will become tired, leading to loss of memory.

"We have discussed the consequences of not following the proper order and principles of treatment according to the four seasons. By utilizing incorrect procedures, one can easily exacerbate a problem. If one does not understand these principles, and correctly remedy the cause of disease, the consequences can be devastating. In diagnosis one should emphasize the precise detection of the nine pulses in the three areas, in order to determine the precise location of the illness. Then render appropriate and effective treatment according to the four seasons so as not to cause chaos to the true qi."

Huang Di said, "I understand."

Qi Bo said, "If one accidentally acupunctures the heart, death will occur within one day. The manifestation will be burping. If one accidentally punctures the liver, death will occur within five days. The symptom will be excessive talking. If one accidentally punctures the lung, death will occur within three days. The symptom will be cough. If one accidentally punctures the kidney, death will occur within six days. The symptom will be sneezing. If one accidentally punctures the spleen, death will occur within ten days. The symptom will be constant swallowing. If one punctures any of the five zang organs, death shall result. By observing the outcome of the treatment, one can accurately predict the prognosis."

CHAPTER 65

—

BIAO AND BEN
AND THE TRANSMISSION
OF DISEASE

—

H UANG DI said, "In disease, there is a differentiation of biao/secondary and ben/primary. In treatment there are effective methods employing the corresponding principles of biao ben or their exact opposing principles. Will you please explain these to me?"

Qi Bo answered, "The principles governing acupuncture treatment dictate that you determine initially whether the illness is yin or yang. Second, you must determine which manifestation came first and which followed. Then you proceed with the treatment. This procedure will make evident whether one should treat according to the corresponding principle or the opposing principle.

"Determine whether to address the biao/secondary or the ben/primary first. It is said that in biao/secondary conditions, one can treat the biao/secondary or the ben/primary depending on the seriousness of the illness. Sometimes one will find that in treating the symptoms, the illness itself can be cured. Sometimes, however, one should ignore the symptoms and treat the root. Sometimes the treatment of correspondence works; other times following the principle of the opposite approach is more effective. Understanding the principle behind this aids one in treatment; not understanding it is a virtual blindness in treatment.

"Yin and yang, determining the disease nature of normal and abnormal and biao/secondary and ben/primary may seem of minor import. But the value of correct application is great, because knowing these principles allows one to know the depth of the disease. Then one can deduce the progression and scope of the illness. The reasoning is quite simple, yet clinically it is difficult to grasp.

"If one suffers from an illness that causes the qi and blood to become chaotic and disharmonious, treat the ben/primary. If the qi and blood were chaotic and disharmonious to begin with, and as a result cause illness, then treat the biao/secondary.

"If a cold pathogen attacks the body, causing a cold condition that creates other pathological changes, treat the cause. If a patient suffers from an illness that manifests as coldness, treat the illness. I know this sounds simple, as if one should treat whatever comes first. But in the clinic how does one really know which precedes?

"If a patient suffers first from febrile disease, which then turns into other pathologic manifestations, treat the original febrile disease. But if a patient has febrile disease first, and then manifests fullness and stagnation in the middle jiao, treat the new symptom first. This is because a stomach that malfunctions cannot absorb food or herbs, and thus any treatment that neglects the stomach is wasted.

"If a patient suffers from an illness and later manifests diarrhea, treat the original illness and then the symptom. If a patient has diarrhea initially and then manifests another illness, treat the cause of diarrhea first. Only then should the manifest illness be treated. If a patient becomes ill and then manifests fullness and obstruction of the middle jiao, treat the fullness and distension—the symptom—immediately. If a patient begins with a full and obstructed middle jiao as the cause, and then manifests restlessness and discomfort of the chest, treat the cause of obstruction immediately. Generally speaking, obstruction of the bowels or urine deserves to be relieved immediately regardless of whether it is a cause or merely a symptom.

"In some cases the patient is attacked by a new pathogen, which causes illness. In other cases, the patient has a preexisting deficiency within the body that may cause the illness. We call the first instance biao/secondary. The second instance we call ben/principle.

"If the pathogen of disease is excess, the condition is excessive. In this case, the pathogen is the ben/primary, while all other symptoms are biao/secondary. First treat the ben/primary, then the biao/secondary. A disease of symptoms that are the result of deficiency of the zheng/antipathogenic qi of the body, the zheng qi deficiency itself is the biao/secondary and the pathogen is the ben/primary. In this case treat the biao/secondary first, then the ben/primary. This will address the deficiency of zheng/antipathogenic qi first. One must be very careful and precise in observing the degree of severity of a condition; then differentiate accordingly the biao/secondary and ben/primary, and which came first. The proper treatment method will be then be easily ascertained.

"When a condition is of a mild nature, one can treat the biao/secondary and ben/primary simultaneously. When a condition is severe, determine a single approach of treating either the ben/primary or the biao/secondary. If one sees obstruction of the bowels or urine, always treat these first.

"In the progression of disease, heart disease will cause heart pain. In one day this will transmit to the lungs, causing cough. By the third day it will transmit to the liver, causing rib pain and distension. In five days it will transmit to the spleen, causing constipation, obstruction, and heaviness of the body. If one does not recover three days after this, death will result. In the winter death occurs in the middle of the night. In summer death occurs at noon.

"In lung disease one suffers dyspnea and cough. Three days later the pathogen will travel to the liver, causing hypochondriac pain and distension. In one day it will transfer to the spleen; this results in muscle pain throughout the body. In five days it transfers to the stomach, leading to epigastric fullness and distension. By the tenth day without healing, death occurs. In the winter death occurs at twilight. In summer death occurs at dawn.

"In liver disease, one suffers from dizziness, vertigo, and hypochondriac fullness. If not healed in three days it transfers to the spleen, causing body aches. In five days it transfers to the stomach, causing abdominal distension. In three more days it transfers to the kidney; this results in back pain, low abdominal pain, and soreness and weakness of the legs. In three more days death will occur. In the winter death occurs at sunset. In the summer death occurs at breakfast.

"In spleen disease one suffers from body ache and heaviness. In one day it transfers to the stomach, causing distension and fullness. In two more days it transfers to the kidneys, causing back pain, low abdominal pain, and soreness in the legs. In three more days it transfers to the bladder, causing spasms and pain along the sides of the spine; obstruction of urine also results. Without healing in ten days, death occurs. In the winter death occurs at the hour of shen or late afternoon. In the summer death occurs at the hour of sunrise.

"In kidney disease one suffers from low abdominal and back pain, and leg soreness and weakness. In three days it transfers to the bladder, causing pain along the spine and urinary obstruction. In three more days it transfers to the stomach, causing abdominal distension. In three more days it transfers to the liver, causing hypochondriac distension and pain. In three more days death will occur. In the winter death occurs at sunrise. In the summer death occurs at twilight.

"In stomach disease one suffers from abdominal pain and distension. In five days it transmits to the kidneys, with the attendant symptoms; in three more days to the bladder; in five more days to the spleen; in six more days death occurs. In the winter death occurs after midnight. In the summer death occurs in the afternoon.

"In disease of the bladder there is pain along the spine and urinary obstruction. In five days the transference is to the kidneys. One day later it transmits to the stomach. One day later it transmits to the spleen. If a cure does not occur within two additional days, death occurs. In the winter death occurs after midnight. In the summer death occurs in the afternoon. This summary reflects the various diseases and their logical progression and transmission. All these illnesses have their definite order of transmission and eventual time of death. One should not use acupuncture in these cases. If, however, the transmission of disease does not follow what we described, if it does not follow the order of progression, one can then utilize acupuncture to effect a cure."

CHAPTER 66

—

ENERGY ALMANAC

—

HUANG DI said, "Under heaven the laws of the five elemental phases are all prevalent. It is represented in the five directions, and brings forth cold, summer heat, dryness, damp, and wind. Within people it is characterized by the five zang organs giving rise to the five qi. In turn the five zang qi manifest the emotions of joy, anger, melancholy, worry, and fear.

"The process of the five elemental phases and their cycle begins on the first day of the year and ends on the last day of the Chinese calendar. The process then repeats over and over. I am now familiar with these theories and principles. But I would like to know the relationships and associations among the five elemental phases and the six atmospheric influences, which affect the three yin and the three yang channels."

One of Huang Di's advisers, Gui Yu Qu, bowed and replied, "This question is very interesting. The five elemental phases and yin and yang are a governing law of the universe. This law exposes the polarities of everything. It outlines the beginning of all transformations of the universe. It governs the growth, development, and eventual destruction of all things.

"Within the dynamic principles lies an intelligence that is difficult to know. The birth and growth of the myriad things we call hua. Growth to the extreme point we call bien. The mysteries of yin and yang are not graspable. We call this shen. To be able to grasp the underlying principles, and to be capable of applying them flexibly, is called sheng. This means sage or wise one.

"The universe potentiates change, which allows all things to manifest and prosper with unlimited energy. It also allows people to have an intelligence with which to understand the logic and reason behind all things. All of this gives rise to the planet Earth, which is able to carry on birth, propagation, and existence. When people reach a deep level of understanding, they become wise. When they become wise, they can truly grasp the boundless potential of energy in the unending interaction of heaven and earth.

"The changes that the universe provides come about in differing forms: in heaven there is wind, on earth there is wood; in heaven there is heat, on earth there is fire; in heaven there is damp, on earth there is earth; in heaven there is dryness, on earth there is metal; in heaven there is cold, on earth there is water. In the heavens there are the six invisible atmospheric influences; on earth there are the visible five elemental phases. The invisible force and the physical forms combine to form the basis for intelligent universal change.

"Heaven and earth are the parameters of the existence of myriad things. Left and right are the paths of the ascending and descending yin and yang. Fire and water, heat and cold symbolize yin and yang. Metal and wood represent the beginning and the end of life. The six atmospheric influences vary, and the five elemental phases are subject to excess and deficiency. Their interaction exposes the nature of excess or deficiency."

Huang Di bowed in turn and said, "I would like to hear you discuss the five elemental phases and their relationship to the seasons."

Gui Yu Qu answered, "The five elemental phases each affects for an entire year. They control more than the four seasons."

Huang Di said, "Will you please elaborate?"

Gui Yu Qu replied, "I have read the sacred book *Tai Shi Tian Yuan Ce* [The Origin of the Universe]. It states that in the vast void of the universe exists the primordial origin of life. The five elemental phases follow the cycles of heaven and combine with the six original cosmic energies that encompass and embrace the entire universe. They set the rhythm for the growth, development, maturation, and death of all things. The nine stars illumine the skies. The seven stars circulate in the solar system. In the circulation of the heavens there is the change of yin and yang. On planet earth there is nurturing and destruction. Day and night contrast with each other. The four seasons have cold and heat. All the myriad things follow this rhythm in their entire life spans. In my family this knowledge has been passed down ten generations. We have researched this wisdom."

Huang Di acknowledged, "Yes. How do you determine if the qi is too much or too little, or if the form is deficient or excess?"

Gui Yu Qu replied, "Yin qi and yang qi have variations in their abundance and insufficiency. That is why we categorize them into three yin and three yang. In terms of form there is deficiency and excess. These describe the five elemental phases as manifested in yearly cycles.

"In ancient times the sages observed the heavens and noted their sur-roundings carefully and proposed a complex system, consisting of several subsystems to account for all possible variables in the forecast of macrocos-mic influences upon the world, especially the weather and the effects on people.

"The basic building blocks of this sytem utilize representative symbols of the ten heavenly stems and the twelve earthly branches, each symbol representing an aspect of natural process. The ten stems in the numerical order of one to ten, with the odd numbers corresponding to yang and the even numbers to yin, is associated with the five elemental phases. If a year is designated as yang it means that the yearly manifestations will tend to be excessive, while yin means that they will tend to be deficient. These stems are, starting with the first stem, jia, the image of breaking through, like a sprout breaking through the earth. It is associated with the wood element and is yang in nature. The second stem, yi, the image of early growth with young and bending stems and branches, corresponds with yin/wood. The third stem, bing, the image of life force expanding like a beautiful bright fire, corresponds with yang/fire. The fourth stem, ding, the image of a new life becoming fully grown, corresponds with yin/fire. The fifth stem, wu, the image of luxuriant growth and prosperous development, corresponds with yang/earth. The sixth stem, ji, the image of distinguishable features and attributes, corresponds with yin/earth. The seventh stem, gen, the image of the beginning of energy reversal, energy retreating until the next spring, corresponds with yang/metal. The eighth stem, xin, the image of withdrawing, corresponds with yin/metal. The ninth stem, ren, the image of the life energy nurtured deeply within, like a pregnant mother nourish-ing the fetus, corresponds with yang/water. And finally the tenth stem, kui, the image of the regathering of a new life force, underground and invisibly cultivated, awaiting a new breakthrough, corresponds to yin/water.

The twelve earthly branches in numerical terms are also divided into six pairs of yin/even and yang/odd classification. They are directly associ-ated with the five elemental phases as well as with the six atmospheric influences and the three yin and three yang steps. The first branch, zi, the image of the reproductiveness of life, like a seed beneath the earth, absorb-ing moisture and nutrition for development, corresponds to yang and water because it is the winter-eleventh month in the Chinese calendar and the hours between eleven P.M. to one A.M. It is associated, however, with the atmospheric influence of imperial fire and shaoyin. The second branch, chou, the image of a sprout before it reaches the surface, or in other words, underground growth, corresponds with yin/earth because it is the twelfth month and the hours between one and three A.M. It is associated with dampness and taiyin. The third branch, yin, the image of a crawling sprout as it meets the warmth of air, its final stretch out of the earth, corresponds with yang/wood because it is the spring first month and the hours between three and five A.M. It is associated with ministerial fire and shaoyang. The fourth branch, mao, the image of luxuriant vegetation dancing in the sunshine, corresponds to yin/wood because it is the second month and the hours between five and seven A.M. It is associated with dryness and yangming. The fifth branch, chen, the image of fully awakening for the coming growth, corresponds with yang/earth because it is the third month of spring or the buffer month between each season and the hours between seven and nine A.M. It is associated with cold and taiyang. The sixth branch, si, the image of the preparation of ripeness, corresponds with yin/fire because it is the summer fourth month and the hours between nine and eleven A.M. It is associated with wind and jueyin. The seventh branch, wu, the image of growth as it reaches its peak, corresponds with yang/fire because it is the fifth month and the hours between eleven A.M. and one P.M. It is associated with imperial fire and shaoyin. The eighth branch, wei, the image of the sweet taste that expresses ripeness and mellowness, corresponds with yin/earth because it is the sixth month and the hours between one and three P.M. It is associated with dampness and taiyin. The ninth branch, shen, the image of the completion of ripeness and the time of harvest, corresponds with yang/metal because it is the autumn/seventh month and the hours between three and five P.M. It is associated with ministerial fire and shaoyang. The tenth branch, you, the image of recollecting after a rich yield, corresponds with yin/metal because it is the eighth month and the hours of five to seven P.M. It is associated with dryness and yangming. The eleventh branch, xu, the image of retreating from the visible excitement of life, corresponds with yang/earth because it is the ninth month and the hours between seven and nine P.M. It is associated with cold and taiyang. The twelfth branch, hai, the image of the seed or core awaiting its next growth, corresponds with yin/water because it is the winter/tenth month and the hours between nine and eleven P.M. It is associated with wind and jueyin."

Huang Di asked, "Will you please explain to me how all of this works?"

Gui Yu Qu answered, "The interactive dynamic between the stems and the branches produces subsystems that make up the large system of meteorology. This sytem is not just about predicting weather patterns but is also about the influence of these weather patterns on all living things in the world, especially people's well-being. It is immensely useful for forecasting epidemic illnesses. In this system we are concerned yearly mainly with three subsystems: the great phase circuit, the host and guest circuit, and the atmospheric influences.

"If the first great circuit is yang or excess, the following circuit will always be yin or deficient. When the great circuit and the ruling atmospheric influence are of the same nature, we call the year tian fu. If the great circuit matches the branch symbol we call the year shui hui. If the great circuit matches the ruling atmospheric influence as well as the branch symbol we call the year san he.

"When the stems and branches are combined, a yang stem can combine only with a yang branch, and a yin stem only with a yin branch, beginning with the combination of jia/zi and ending with kui/hai. This gives a total of sixty possible combinations, which are used to denote the sixty-year and sixty-day cycles. The ancients observed that in nature, patterns at large repeated itself every sixty years, and thus at the end of the sixtieth year the cycle started all over again. Each year in the Chinese calendar is divided into twenty-four fortnightly segments called jie qi or solar terms. Four terms equal sixty days and is called a bu or step. Six steps makes up a year. In a sixty-year cycle there are all together 1,440 solar terms.

"Cold, summer heat, dryness, dampness, wind, and fire represent the yin and the yang of the heavens. They correspond to the three yin and the three yang. Wood, fire, metal, earth, and water represent the yin and the yang of the earth. They correspond to the changes of the universe. Heaven came from the birth of yang, the sustenance of yin. In nature the yang can be destructive while the yin is protective. If you truly want to know about the yin and the yang of heaven and earth, you must understand how the six atmospheric influences interact with the five elemental phases. This interaction brings about changes in weather, nature, disease, and healing."

Huang Di said, "What the Master has conveyed includes the secrets of heaven and earth. It has been very clear and I will remember forever what I have heard today. This way I will be better able to relieve the suffering of my citizens and govern my health. I will teach my citizens so that they understand these principles. I hope to transmit this from generation to generation so people of the future will have fewer worries."

Gui Yu Qu said, "The five elemental phases and the six atmospheric influences have a definite pattern and rhythm. This knowledge is very profound. If one grasps it, one can know the changes that will transpire in the natural world. One who masters this science can enjoy eternal health. One who neglects to learn this will suffer danger, injury, and even death by having violated the natural rhythms and patterns of the universe. Please learn, understand, and apply this knowledge carefully."

Huang Di said, "In order to understand this deeply, one must know its origin and consequences. Then one will know the near and the far. In this fashion, the understanding and application of the five elemental phases and the six atmospheric influences will enable one to achieve clarity. Is it possible for you to summarize this in a simple form so that we can more easily understand and recall it?"

Gui Yu Qu answered, "You ask very meaningful questions. The wisdom will become apparent to you very quickly. It is like hitting the drum and hearing the sound; it is like the echo that results from speaking. It is that transparent; it is that simple."

Huang Di replied, "This is illuminating. You have communicated in a specific manner. I will carve it on a jade tablet and preserve it in the *Golden Chamber,* and I will call it 'Discussion on the Cosmos.' "

CHAPTER 67

THE FIVE-PHASE CIRCUITS

—

HUANG DI consulted Qi Bo while attempting to organize the body of the knowledge of cosmology. He asked, "I've been in discussion with Gui Yu Qu about the yearly energetic phases according to the heavenly stems and the earthly branches. He mentioned that in the sixty-year cycle the jia/ji stem years are governed by the earth phase, the yi/gen by metal, bing/xin by water, ding/ren by wood, and finally wu/kui by fire. Similarly, the zi/wu branch years are ruled by the Imperial Fire and correspond to shaoyin, chou/wei by dampness, earth, and taiyin, yin/shen by ministerial fire and shaoyang, mao/you by dryness, metal, and yangming, chen/xu by cold, water, and taiyang, and last, si/hai by wind, wood, and jueyin. My confusion lies in how they came to be phases and the six atmospheric influences. Could you enlighten me?"

Qi Bo answered, "This resulted from countless years of observation of the natural world by the ancient sages, who then classified these changes into a workable framework that is in concert with the prevailing universal laws of yin/yang and the five elemental phases."

Huang Di asked again, "Can you please explain to me the origins of this system of phase energetics?"

Qi Bo answered, "You've asked a very pertinent question. In order to understand the origin of the phase energetic system, one must possess knowledge of astronomy. I've referred to the classic *Tai Shi Tian Yuan Ce* in the past for this information. The planets within our galaxy exert the most influence on phenomena in our world. There are further twenty-eight constellations that are observable to the naked eye in the heavens that also are significant in their import to human life. The constellations also span the entire sky, adding up to 360 degrees. With the North Star as the center of the circle in the sky, one can identify the four directions and hence each of the corresponding groups of constellations. Starting with the eastern seven constellations shaped like a dragon they are Jiao, the Horn;

Keng, the Neck; Di, the Bottom, Fang, the House; Xin, the Heart; Wei, the Tail, and Ji, the Basket. The northern seven constellations shaped like a turtle are as follows: Dou, the Pipe; Niu, the Ox; Nu, the Maiden; Xu, the Void; Wei, the Crisis; Shi, the Room; and Bi, the Wall. The western seven constellations shaped like a tiger are as follows: Kui, the Champion; Lou, the Hump; Wei, the Stomach; Mao, the Rooster's Crown; Bi, the Fark; Zu, the Beak; and Shen, the Interwoven. The southern seven con-stellations shaped like a bird are as follows: Jing, the Well; Gui, the Ghost; Liu, the Willow; Xin, the Star; Zhang, the Drawn Bow; Yi, the Wing; and Zhen, the Carriage. Five energetic colors can be seen from the interactive movement of the constellations that corresponds to the five elemental phases. For example, red can be observed bridging the northern Niu and Nu with the western Kui constellation. Yellow can be observed bridging the eastern Xin and Wei with the southern Zhen constellations. Green can be observed bridging the Northern Wei and Shi with the southern Liu and Gui constellations. White can be observed bridging eastern Kang and Di with the western Mao and Bi constellations. Black can be observed bridg-ing southern Zhang and Yi with the Lei and Wei constellations. Knowing the movement of the heavenly bodies and its relationship and import to the natural world is the first step to understand the rudiments of the phase energetic system."

Huang Di acknowledged Qi Bo's response and asked, "I've heard Gui Yu Qu remark that the heaven is the top and earth is the bottom that contain the myriad things, while to the left and right are the space that allows for the transformation of yin and yang to take place. What exactly does he mean?"

Qi Bo replied, "This has to do with the yearly cycle of the atmo-sphereic influences. Each year there is a primary influence that affects mainly the first half of the year and that then rotates among the six influ-ences in a given order in the years following. For convenience, imagine a wheel with the dominant influence at the top, or north, opposite the sec-ondary influence at the bottom or south, which affects the last half of the year, and to the left and right are the other influence in order. For instance, if the primary influence of a given year is wind/jueyin at the top of the wheel, in relation to the top, to the left would be imperial fire/shaoyin and to the right would be cold/taiyang. Similarly if one finds the secondary influence ministerial fire/shaoyang at the bottom, in relation to the bottom,

to the left would be dryness/yangming and to the right would be damp-
ness/taiyin.

When the primary atmospheric influence of a year is in harmony with
the great circuit of that year, that is, when the influence is in a creative
phase in relation to the circuit, for example, wood versus fire, then the
weather patterns and disease will be milder. On the contrary, disharmony
results if the influence is in a control phase in relation to the circuit, thus
overpowering the normally expected patterns to give rise to dramatic and
extreme shifts in weather and disease."

Huang Di asked, "How do the six atmospheric influences affect the
earth?"

Qi Bo replied, "The seasons change with the six atmospheric influences giving rise to the birth, growth, decline, and death of all things in
nature. Dryness withers, summer heat/ministerial fire increases the temperature, wind promotes movement, dampness moistens, cold freezes, and
fire/imperial fire hardens the earth."

Huang Di asked, "Can one detect the primary and secondary atmo-
sphereic influences in a person's pulses?"

Qi Bo replied, "No, the yearly influences are not directly detectable
in one's pulses. However, each seasonally normal pulse patterns should ob-
viously reflect the influence of that given season. If the pulse patterns do
not follow this natural occurrence and instead manifest out-of-order patterns, then the prognosis will certainly be poor."

Huang Di asked, "Can you explain further the relationshp between
the six atmospheric influences and that of people and their environment?

Qi Bo answered, "The influences play an important role in nature.
They bring about transformation in everything on earth, including people.
There is nothing that is untouched by the six atmospheric changes. Let me
tell about them individually.

"In the east, wind arises, there is movement that promotes green
woody growth, and when unripe, gives off a sour taste. The sour taste
stimulates the liver when ingested and nourishes the tendons and ligaments.
When the wind is gentle it harmonizes all, but when it is extreme it can be
destructive, just as in people, emotion turns into rage when the liver is out
of control. Metal is the control element, so therefore grief counters anger
while dryness lessens the wind and pungent neutralizes sour.

"In the south, red flame and summer heat arise causing abundant
growth and development, but when extreme they burn things down and

give off a scorched bitter taste. The bitter taste stimulates the heart and circulation. When the fire is controlled it increases productivity, but when it goes out of control, people become overly excited, which can bring harm to the heart. Water is the control element, so therefore terror, salty, and cold can counter overexcitment, bitter taste, and fire, respectively.

"In the center, damp and yellowing mud provides rich nourishment that ripens vegetation, giving off a sweet taste that stimulates the spleen and nourishes the flesh. In harmony it promotes quiet contentment, but in extreme situations emotional manifestations occur that can be wearying to the spleen. Wood is the controlling element, so therefore anger, wind, and sourness can counter worry, dampness, and sweetness, respectively.

"In the west, dryness is prevalent through the desert mountains that contain a wealth of metal ore and vegetation that is pungent to the tongue. The pungent taste invigorates the lungs and opens the pores. In harmony it promotes calmness while in extremes it withers and destroys prematurely. Sadness is common to it, which weakens the lungs. Fire is the controlling element, so therefore excitement and bitter can counter sadness and pungent, respectively.

"In the north, the massive glaciers and deep dark seas give rise to coldness and a salty taste from the ocean. The salty taste stimulates the kidney and nourishes the bones and inspires fear in people. In harmony it provides quietude but in extremes it causes great freezes and hailstorms that destroy. Fear and salty can be overcome by reasoning and bitter, which are the attributes of its controlling element, the fire.

Huang Di asked, "What is the relationship between the timing of these influences and the prognosis of disease?"

Qi Bo answered, "When the atmospheric influences follow the natural order of appearance, illness can be easily rectified. When the contrary occurs, rehabilitation of illness will be difficult."

CHAPTER 68

THE SIX ATMOSPHERIC
INFLUENCES

H UANG DI asked, "The law that governs the movement of the heavenly bodies and the six atmospheric influences is profound and significant. Can you tell me more about its practical application?"

Qi Bo replied, "In regard to the six atmospheric influences, there is a
definitive order governing their appearance on a yearly and seasonal basis.
We have spoken in the past about the yearly ruling influences that set the
general weather trend for the first and last half of the year and that also
dictate the weather patterns for each season. Any violation of this rhythm
would bring about excess or deficient states.

"The six influences of cold, fire, dryness, dampness, heat, and wind
are referred to as the ben or primary aspect. The three yang and the three
yin channels of taiyang, shaoyang, yangming, taiyin, shaoyin, and jueyin
are referred to as the biao or secondary aspect of the six influences. The ben
originates in the cosmos while the biao manifests on earth. For instance, fire
is the ben while shaoyang is the biao as well as its primary ruling influence,
and jueyin is its secondary ruling influence.

"Ben and biao each will have different disease indications, despite
their association, depending upon which is the dominant influence at a
given time and thus exerts the greatest impact."

Huang Di asked, "Why is it that sometimes the seasonal atmospheric
influence appears in concert with the start of each season and other times
the atmospheric influence appears either too soon or too late?"

Qi Bo replied, "It is dependent on the excess or deficient nature of
the primary ruling atmospheric influence of that year."

Huang Di asked, "What are the consequences to disease during these
years of imbalance in the circuits and influences?"

Qi Bo replied, "When the elemental phase of a great circuit matches that of the earthly branches, it is called a sui hui year. When the phase of a great circuit matches that of the yearly primary ruling influence, it is called a tian fu year. When the phase matches that of the branch and ruling influence, it is called a tai yi tian fu year. During a shui hui year, diseases are likely to be acute and severe; a tian fu year will typically bring on diseases more gradually and less severe, whereas in a tai yi tian fu year the diseases are likely to be violent and usually end in death."

Huang Di asked, "How do the five elemental phases interact with the six atmospheric influences on a yearly and seasonal basis?"

Qi Bo replied, "First the heavenly stem shall determine the phase of the great circuit of the given year, then the earthly branch combined with the stem shall determine the yearly and seasonal ruling primary and secondary influences. The twenty-four solar terms of a year are divided into six steps of four terms each. Each step is about slightly more than sixty days long and is governed by an atmospheric influence. The first step consists of four terms of beginning of spring, rain water, waking from hibernation, and spring equinox. The second step consists of four terms of clear and bright, rain for grains, beginning of summer, and budding grain. The third step consists of four terms of bearded grain, summer solstice, slight heat, and great heat. The fourth step consists of beginning of autumn, limited heat, white dew, and autumnal equinox. The fifth step consists of four terms of cold dew, hoarfrost, beginning of winter, and mild snow. The sixth and last step consists of four terms of heavy snow, winter solstice, slight cold, and severe cold.

"The arrival time of each atmospheric influence in each step differs during different circuit years. For instance, during jia/zi year the first step begins on the first hour of severe cold and ends sixty days and fourteen and a half hours later on spring equinox. The second step begins following the first step and goes also the same amount of time to budding grain. The third step begins immediately and ends on great heat. The fourth step starts and ends on autumnal equinox. The fifth step ends on mild snow. And the sixth step ends at four hours and ten minutes on the first day of severe cold. This completes the three hundred and sixty degrees of the earth encircling the sun in one revolution. In the following yi/chou year the first step would start from the ending time of the sixth step of jia/zi year. This cycle continues for every year afterward. The ending time is the same for the years of yin, wu, and xu; mao, wei, and hai; chen, shen and zi; and si, you, and chou."

Huang Di asked, "What causes the natural atmospheric influences to become pathogenic?"

Qi Bo replied, "The natural cyclic movement of the universe makes possible the birth, growth, decline, and death of all things. By the same token, any variation to this cyclic movement will produce imbalance, which in turn is reflected as a pathogenic threat to living beings."

Huang Di asked, "Are there any persons who are not affected by the pathogenic influences?"

Qi Bo replied, "You have asked a very special question. It is not possible for ordinary beings to escape the effects of the atmospheric influences. However, only the immortals and highly achieved beings who merge their beings as one with the universe are exempt from the effects of the atmospheric influences."

CHAPTER 69

—

EFFECTS OF THE FIVE ELEMENTAL PHASES AND THE SIX ATMOSPHERIC INFLUENCES

—

HUANG DI said, "As the six atmospheric influences of nature and the five elemental phases of earth interact, a cycle of changes is produced that is relatively consistent. Summer follows spring, winter follows autumn, and so on. The yin and yang oscillate and manifest throughout the universe. This is a delicate balance that has a tendency to become disordered. Nature has a method of putting things back in order, but the tendency toward irregularity never ceases. As a result, some of the qi and blood of the six channels becomes disrupted. The original qi of the five zang organs moves in a dynamic way whereas some qi becomes dominant and other qi becomes deficient. I would like to understand the reasons behind this and their rhythm."

Qi Bo answered, "You have asked a very good question. You should understand this because this question has been asked by emperors for generations. The wisdom has been passed down by teachers of medicine for generations. My knowledge is shallow, but I have heard my teacher discussing these issues."

Huang Di said, "It has been stated that if one finds the worthy student but does not teach him, the result is shi dao, or loss of the knowledge. This harms the transmission of knowledge. On the other hand, if one teaches the wisdom to inappropriate students, this is an expression of irresponsibility. I myself do not fit the criteria of the most ideal student. But I am compassionate toward my citizens and want to relieve them of their suffering. Therefore, I would like you, Master, to pass this knowledge on to me for the sake of future generations. I will conform to the ethics and requirements of the tradition."

Qi Bo replied, "Very well. In the book *Shang Jing* (Classic of Medicine) it is said that one who studies medicine must understand the knowledge of the universe—cosmology. One must also understand the geography and geology of the earth, including the five elements. One also needs to know and understand people. Only in this way can one have a complete understanding of medicine."

Huang Di asked, "Can you speak in more detail?"

Qi Bo said, "These understandings are important and necessary in order to determine the position of heaven in relation to earth and to people. This will enable one to perceive all normal and abnormal movements. Knowing the normal and abnormal movements of heaven and earth, one can readily know and anticipate the same movements within mankind. This enables the physician to more effectively treat disease, and more importantly, to prevent it. To know the natural way, one must continually cultivate one's true nature. Knowing the natural way, of course, allows one to also understand the unnatural way."

Huang Di said, "In the five elemental phases, what is it that occurs in conditions of excess?"

Qi Bo replied, "When a wood phase year is excess, there will be strong wind. The spleen, or earth element, will suffer damage. In this situation people often suffer indigestion, diarrhea, loss of appetite, heavy limbs, lethargy, repressed emotions, borborygmus, and distension and fullness of the abdomen. This is because the wood energy is too strong. You will observe that the corresponding planet in our solar system is very bright. This planet, Sui/Jupiter, indicates that the wood energy is excessive. That is why the ancient Taoists looked to the heavens for answers; it allowed them to determine what was going to happen to people or society. The excess wood also affects human beings by causing anger, dizziness, vertigo, and diseases of the head. This describes earth energy being weakened by the wood energy. It is like the clouds in the sky racing past; a frantic movement of the myriad things on earth, vegetation shaking and trees falling. Patients display hypochondriac pain and ceaseless vomiting. When the pulse on the stomach channel on the foot near the chongyang (ST42) point cannot be detected, the indication is often an incurable disease. In the heavens, we see another star that brightens, Tai Bu/Venus, the metal planet. This signifies that as the wood is excess, metal energy has begun to rise, in an attempt to control it.

"When a fire phase year becomes excessive, heat becomes extreme, causing injury to the lung. People suffer from malaria, difficulty breathing, cough, wheezing, dyspnea, vomiting of blood, nosebleeds, blood in the urine and bowel movements, watery diarrhea, difficulty swallowing, dry throat, deafness, and feverish sensation in the chest, shoulder, or upper back. Here the metal is dominated by fire energy and is in a state of decline. In this instance, when we look to the heavens, we see that the fire planet, Ronghuo/Mars, is very bright, indicating that the fire energy is excessive. In disease one finds chest pain, distension and fullness of the hypochondrium, rib pain, pain between the chest and shoulder, pain on the inside of the arms, fever, and body aches. When the fire energy is excessive, nature will manifest rain, frost, and freezing. This indicates that the extreme fire has transmitted to the water energy. In heaven we can observe the water planet, Chen/Mercury, shining more brightly. If we encounter a year that is affected by either shaoyin or shaoyang, fire becomes even worse. Drought results, and people manifest delirium, spasms, mania, convulsions of the extremities, cough, dyspnea, difficulty breathing, bleeding from the lower body, and uncontrollable diarrhea and urination. If the radial pulse at taiyuan (LU9) is undetectable, death will follow shortly. In the heavens, Mars shines brightly.

"When the earth phase energy is excess, weather patterns become damp and rainy. The pathogen affects the kidneys. People complain of abdominal pain, coldness in the extremities, suppressed emotions, melancholy, heaviness of the body, restlessness, and irritability. Atrophy of the flesh and muscles occurs to the point where one cannot walk. There are spasms and pain, swelling, and edema, a decrease in appetite, and weak limbs. All this is because the earth element is diseased. In the heavens, we can see that the earth planet, Zheng/Saturn, is very bright. In nature, when earth is excessive damp prevails. Springs rush from the earth; floods occur. When the wood energy is involved there are severe storms, tornados, and typhoons; dams burst. People suffer from swollen and distended abdomens, ascites, diarrhea, and borborygmus. If we find that the taixi (K3) pulse by the ankle is undetectable, death is indicated.

"In a year where the metal phase is excessive, dryness is prevalent. The pathogen invades the liver. People suffer from abdominal and hypochondriac pain, redness and ulceration of the eyes, and difficulty hearing. When dryness is strong the body is heavy and there is chest pain, irritability, pain radiating to the back, distension in the ribs, and pain in the low abdomen. The metal planet, Tai Bu/Venus, is brightly illuminated. Within the human body there is difficulty breathing, dyspnea, shoulder pain, and pain in the joints. The metal energy is strong, but the fire energy is also very strong. Thus Mars increases in brightness. If the metal energy suddenly becomes excessive, causing a decline in wood energy, then vegetation becomes wilted and fails to grow. People suffer from sudden pain in the ribs, difficulty turning, cough, dyspnea, vomiting of blood, and nosebleeds. If the taichong (LIV3) pulse on the foot is undetectable, the condition is incurable. Tai Bu/Venus, the metal planet, is exceptionally bright.

"When water energy is excessive, cold energy becomes prevalent and the pathogen attacks the heart. Patients will manifest fever, palpitations, irritability, cold extremities, cold body, delirium, and chest pain. When the cold energy arrives too early, the water planet, Chen/Mercury, is very bright in the sky. Excess of the water pathogen causes water retention in the abdomen, swelling in the feet, cough, and dyspnea, wheezing, night sweats, and aversion to wind. In this case, the wood energy begins to exert its influence, causing a downpour of rain and fog. The earth planet, Zheng/Saturn, becomes brighter. In the years controlled by taiyang energy the weather patterns are of strong rain, hail, freezing, and snow. Dampness causes changes in all things. People have distension in the abdomen, borborygmus, diarrhea with undigested food, and extreme thirst. If the shenmen (H7) pulse on the wrist is undetectable, death is inevitable. The planet Ronghuo/Mars will be dimly illuminated, while Chen/Mercury will be very bright."

Huang Di said, "Thank you. Now will you please tell me about the deficiencies of the five elemental phases?"

Qi Bo answered, "You ask very detailed questions. In a year where the wood phase is weak, the dry energy becomes excessive. If the yearly energy does not correspond to growth, vegetation does not proliferate; in fact, vegetation becomes malnourished and wilts quickly. Ronghuo/Mars is very bright. Patients suffer from middle jiao qi deficiency and coldness. There is hypochondriac pain, low abdominal pain, borborygmus, and diarrhea. Weather patterns are of cold rain. In the five grains, green-colored grain does not ripen but stays green. If yangming governs the year, metal energy inhibits the wood. The wood energy then loses its nature of thrusting and growth. Vegetation does not become luxuriant until summer and autumn. Spring growth is bypassed; thus, the period of bearing fruit is short and hurried. Plants and vegetation wilt and die early. The metal and earth stars are dominant in the heavens.

Metal energy overcontrols the wood; this causes wood to give birth to fire. The resulting heat dominates and turns what is moist to dryness and what is tender to brittleness. There is a quick stage of maturation and fruit-bearing. Blossoming and fruit-bearing actually occur simultaneously. Patients suffer from heat; there is stagnation under the skin. Symptoms are fever and chills, boils, carbuncles and various skin conditions, acne, and hemorrhoids. The metal and fire stars are bright. Grains are dry and brittle and not abundant. Frost comes early in this year. This causes strange cold spells and rain, which damage the crops. Foods that tend to be yellow and sweet in taste will suffer spoilage and insect invasion. This is a bad year for harvest. The earth element of the spleen is more easily invaded by pathogens. This is followed by fire energy, which overcontrols metal. Because metal energy is weakened it cannot encourage crops to ripen as usual in the autumn. Patients suffer from cough and congestion of the nose. The fire and metal planets are brightest.

"When the year of the fire phase is deficient, cold energy dominates. The summer season alters; all things in nature lack the support of prosperous development. Cold yin energy stagnates and suppresses yang qi, which then cannot transform all things to cause maturation. Chen/Mercury is brighter than usual. Patients suffer chest pain, hypochondriac distension, pain in the upper back between the shoulder blades, and pain along the inner arm. The qi rebels upward, causing vertigo, dizziness, chest pain, sudden loss of voice, swelling in the chest and abdomen, and pain in the low back that radiates to the ribs. The limbs may be weak, tired, contracted, and unable to straighten. The thigh and hip become stiff. Ronghuo/Mars becomes dim, while Chen/Mercury becomes bright. The red-colored crops do not ripen. Fire has been overcontrolled by water. This leads to earth energy rising; there is then an enormous downpour of rain. The earth energy then attempts to control water; thus, we find diarrhea, abdominal distension and pain, lack of appetite, coldness in the middle jiao, borborygmus, and spasms of the feet with numbness and difficulty walking. Zheng/Saturn now becomes bright, while Chen/Mercury becomes dim. Dark grains and crops have trouble ripening.

"In a year that is deficient in the earth phase, the wind energy rises and the earth energy loses its transformational properties. When the wind energy is abundant, there is prosperous growth of vegetation. However, because transformational energy is lacking, all things appear to be growing but are not solid. Sui/Jupiter is bright in the sky. People manifest indigestion, diarrhea, vomiting, cholera, heavy body, abdominal pain, twitching of the tendons, creakiness of the bones, soreness, and pain of the muscles; they are also susceptible to anger. The cold water energy is not controlled and arises. Insects and animals go into early hibernation. People suffer coldness in the middle jiao. Sui/Jupiter is bright and Zheng/Saturn is dim. Yellow crops and vegetation do not ripen. Wood may suppress the earth; the earth reacts by supporting the metal element. Weather patterns of autumn emerge; strong vibrant trees lose their leaves and their energy returns to the root. People experience acute spastic pain of the rib area that radiates to the low abdomen, and shortness of breath. Sweet yellow crops are consumed by insects. When the pathogen affects the earth element, people suffer lack of appetite. When the metal energy becomes strong enough to control the wood, the green-colored crops suffer. The metal star is now bright, while the earth star dims. In jueyin years the ministerial fire is prevalent. The normal deep freeze does not take place; and insects that are supposed to be hibernating begin to be active again.

"The earth is aided by fire and this prevents wood from dominating the earth. In this case, Sui/Jupiter shines brightly above and people are generally disease free during this time.

"In a year of deficiency of metal, fire and wood are vibrant. The energy from the late summer rises to an excess state. All things then become very strong. The weather turns very dry and hot. Ronghuo/Mars is very bright at this time. People often suffer from heaviness and tension of the shoulder and back, nasal congestion, sneezing, blood in the stools, and acute diarrhea. The consolidating energy of autumn does not arrive on time. This causes the metal star to become very dim. White-colored crops do not ripen on time. The fire pathogen suppresses metal. Metal then causes water to arise. This leads to sudden cold rain, hail, and snow, which destroy things and cause the yin qi to become so extreme that it pushes the yang upward. People suffer fever and pain in the head radiating to the neck. In the sky Chen/Mercury becomes very bright. Red-colored crops do not properly ripen. People also have ulcers, mouth sores, and chest pain.

"In a year of deficiency of water, the damp earth qi is dominant. Water cannot control fire, and fire becomes blazing. The weather is very hot with intermittent rain. The transformation of the myriad things speeds up; the earth star is very bright. People often suffer from abdominal distension, fullness, heaviness of body, diarrhea, yin-type boil and carbuncle conditions, abscesses with watery discharge, low back and hip pain, joint stiffness of the lower extremities, irritability, suppressed emotions, and weakness and atrophy of the legs, coldness, pain in the bottom of the feet, and swelling in the top. All these conditions are due to the hidden energy of the winter being unable to exercise its function; the kidney qi is balanced. Chen/Mercury loses its brightness. Black-colored crops do not ripen properly. In a year governed by taiyin the cold water energy dominates. This causes all water on the planet to freeze. Hibernation comes early. Yang energy becomes hidden and cannot exercise its warming action. People manifest lower body coldness, abdominal swelling, and water retention. Saturn is bright and the yellow crops ripen. The earth pathogen overcontrols the water, which in turn creates wood rising. This prompts severe windstorms to destroy vegetation. In people, the power to grow properly is diminished. The facial complexion changes frequently, there are spasms and pain of the tendons, difficulty moving, spasms of the muscles, blurry vision or blindness; things look cracked; there are various wind skin rashes. If the pathogen enters the chest and disphragm, there is chest or abdominal pain. This is all due to the wood energy becoming excessive; the earth energy has been damaged or suppressed. The crops that correspond to wood will not ripen properly. Sui/Jupiter becomes very bright."

Huang Di said, "Thank you very much for that answer. Will you please now tell me the relationship between the five elemental phases and the four seasons?"

Qi Bo replied, "You have asked another important question that requires quite a detailed answer. If the year of the wood is in decline, and if in the spring there is sufficient wind to enable fertilization of vegetation, in the autumn there will be dewdrops and normal cool weather. If in the spring we see severe cold and frost, the summer will bring extreme heat. Disruptive patterns will manifest in the eastern direction, and in people, in the liver and hypochondriac area, and in the tendons and joints. In the year where fire is in decline, if the summer has normal weather the winter will also have normal cold trends. If the summer is abnormally cold, the late summer will be very wet. The pattern of destruction will manifest in the southerly direction. In people this means the heart, chest and channels will be affected.

"In the year where earth is in decline, if there is a mild, dusty wind with a drizzle in the third, sixth, ninth, and twelfth months, we consider this normal. When spring comes there will be a mild wind and warming trend. However, if in the latter part of each of the aforementioned months there is a severe wind that overturns trees, rain, frost, and snow will be dominant in the autumn. The pattern of destruction manifests in the four extremities and spleen, also in the epigastrium.

"In a year of deficiency of metal, if there is normal weather in the summer, the winter will be normal too. But if the summer is excessively hot, the autumn will bring hail, frost, and snow. Its pattern of destruction is the westerly direction; in people, this is in the lungs. The location of disease is the chest, hypochondriac area, shoulders, upper back, and skin.

"In a year of deficiency of water, if there are dusty windstorms during the third, sixth, ninth, and twelfth months, trees will fall as a result. The destructive pattern is of the northern direction; in people, destruction is in the kidneys. The locations of disease are the back, spine, and bone marrow. The muscles and behind the knees will also be affected.

"The five elemental phases are always in a delicate balance. Control must be applied to excess; assistance must be provided for decline. When normal things are rhythmic and peaceful the four seasons also have their rhythm. When this rhythm is lost, energy of heaven and earth becomes chaotic. Stagnation and extreme weather patterns result. The active and passive actions of nature are controlled by the regulating functions of heaven and earth."

Huang Di said, "The master's exposition on the five elemental phase cycles in relation to the four seasons has been very detailed. I am grateful for this. However, I also have questions about the chaotic patterns that arise. They do not have a predetermined pattern; how then does one know what to expect?"

Qi Bo replied, "The changes of the five elemental phases, although not always predictable, can be determined by observing the changing phenomena on earth."

Huang Di asked, "Will you please tell me more about this?"

Qi Bo answered, "Wind comes from the east and promotes the rising of wood energy. The nature of wood is dispersing, softening, and harmonizing. It is responsible for causing germination and opening the flow of yang qi. This moves through the tendons and luo. When abnormal it disperses excessively or is not stable. When destructive, it kills.

"Heat arises from the south and brings about an abundance of fire. The nature of fire is brightness and exhibition. It promotes a proper vibrant development. It illuminates and displays prosperity of all things. When it varies and becomes abnormal it tends to burn, concentrate, and exhaust.

"Dampness manifests in the middle. It assists the earth energy in becoming strong. Its uniqueness is in its lubricating function. It solidifies all things: crops, trees, fruits. It is quieting and calm, but when it undergoes change we see sudden rainstorms and downpours that are strong enough to destroy dams.

"Dryness arises from the west. It can enhance metal energy, which is clean, uninhibited and bold. In nature dryness shrinks and solidifies. When it changes all things become more contracted. When it becomes destructive things wilt and die.

"Coldness flows from the north. It supports the water energy. Water is cold, clear, calm, and secretive. It has depth. It functions to consolidate, coagulate, and solidify. When it changes, severe cold and freezing occur. It causes strong snowstorms.

"When observing the nature and changes of these different energies, their uniqueness, manifestations, transformational properties, and destructive tendencies can all be noted. Then one can grasp the changes of the myriad things in nature. One can also comprehend the causes of disease in man."

Huang Di said, "You have talked about the five energies, their excesses, and their deficiencies. These correspond with the five planets mentioned previously. If all these patterns become nonrhythmic and destructive, and if the changes are sudden, will this be reflected in the planets too?"

Qi Bo answered, "The five elemental planets follow the flow of the universe as they move. They always move according to a set pattern and rhythm that reflects the norm. Sudden changes that occur on earth may be due to other phenomena and do not affect the pathway of the planets."

Huang Di asked, "How are the five planets affected by the energy cycles?"

Qi Bo replied, "They move and rotate according to the great universal energy cycle."

Huang Di said, "The planets travel in specific paths and at given speeds. Can you explain this to me?"

Qi Bo answered, "When the five planets seem to linger, their illumination will decrease. This is because they are in observation of the human world. If the planets travel quickly over an archway and then seem to reverse their course, it is because they are aware of people's virtues and sins. If the planets linger along their pathways for a long time it is because they are ready to bestow benevolence upon the virtuous and disaster upon the sinners.

"How do these variations affect energy and weather patterns in nature? They have their largest impact when the planet is closest to earth, and their smallest impact when a planet is farther away. When the illumination is twice as bright as normal there is an abundance of energy. When the illumination is three times as bright, benevolence and disaster will strike soon. If illumination is one-half as bright, the energy impact will decrease. If illumination is one-quarter as bright, the impact is minimal from the planets.

"There is always a planet among the five elemental planets that corresponds to a given year's energy cycle. If a year is one of excess the planet will leave its normal path when traveling in the northern direction. The planet will also lose some of its brightness. In a year of depletion the planet will have a tinge of color that corresponds to the controlling element. If a year is harmonious the planets will follow their normal paths. One who is keen in observing the universe should be able to observe these aforementioned changes and prepare accordingly for shifts in energy. One who does not make these observations will misguide the leaders of their communities."

Huang Di said, "Will you please explain more about disasters?"

Qi Bo answered, "This all derives from changes in energy; sometimes there may be excess and other times, deficiency. Disasters are contingent upon a confluence of time and circumstance. One must observe the cycles of the planets to know these factors."

Huang Di said, "What is considered a disastrous response, and what is considered favorable?"

Qi Bo replied, "Happiness, health, and peacefulness are the favorable responses while anger, disease, and restlessness are negative responses. One can observe the planets to know when one's fortune will change."

Huang Di asked, "Is it the changes in the placement of the planets that induce these responses?"

Qi Bo answered, "In regard to the placement of the planets, the responses are accurate and the impact to people is the same."

Huang Di said, "Thank you for your enlightenment. How do the five elemental phases affect people and the myriad things in nature?"

Qi Bo replied, "The energy cycles follow specific universal law and will exert predictable influence on people and nature."

Huang Di said, "What is their relationship to disease?"

Qi Bo replied, "The constructive energy cycle promotes growth and health, and the destructive cycle promotes death and disease. In man, antipathogenic qi defends against pathogenic qi. Then the antipathogenic qi becomes passive and unable to defend, illness is the result. If one is invaded by more pathogenic qi, the illness deepens."

Huang Di said, "Thank you for your explanation. What you have communicated to me are profound philosophies and principles. These are great works of ancient sages who devoted their entire lifetimes to learning and understanding. I have heard that one who understands the heavens will also understand people. One who understands ancient times shall understand the present. One who has a firm grasp of energy transformations will also understand the myriad things. One who knows how to adapt to the environment will take advantage of the cycles of the universe. One who understands transformation and change will understand the essence of nature. You have these understandings, Master. Other than you, who could teach this rarified knowledge? I must choose an auspicious day to record and store these teachings in my library. Every morning I will study them and I shall call them 'The Transformational Properties of Cosmic Energies.'

"Further, I shall treasure this information and will be most selective about whom I pass it on to."

CHAPTER 70

—

RULES OF PHASE ENERGETICS

—

H UANG DI said, "Within the sixty-year cycle each yearly circuit manifests differently in nature and in people, depending on whether it is in a state of harmony, excess, or deficiency. I would like to hear you discuss these variations."

Qi Bo replied, "I will try to answer you in as detailed a fashion as possible. Generally, during normal or harmonious phase years, the weather patterns and their effects on people follow a normal course and reflect neither extreme. During excess years the excess elemental energy exerts unduly effects upon nature and people, creating extreme conditions, and the end result is often catastrophic. During deficient years the elemental energy is unable to exercise its characteristic power, and it therefore contributes to a decline in normal activities in nature and in people. I will now discuss each specific phase year and its variations.

"In a wood phase year, a harmonious year is characterized by the balanced wood elemental attributes of balmy weather, prevalance of vegetation, natural activites in ceaseless motion. In people the liver, upper abdomen, and eyes are the site of disease.

"An excess year is characterized by a profusion of wood attributes that may bring great windstorms that damage new plantings and that uproot trees in spring. Disease of the liver, gallbladder, spleen, and stomach and their corresponding channels as well as dizziness, shaking, rage, and pain in the vertex of one's head are common afflictions during this time. If the yearly ruling primary influence is shaoyang/fire or shaoyin/heat, the fire fueled by the excess wood in the creative cycle in turn becomes forceful, leading to vomiting of blood and mania. Furthermore, dysfunction of the digestion becomes prevalent as the earth phase is overcontrolled by the excess wood. Finally, when autumn arrives it is likely to be particularly harsh, and rapid decline in nature would be obvious. At this time, one's liver is particularly vulnerable to illness.

"A deficient year is characterized by a shortage of wood attributes that may bring a cool, dark climate in the spring that stalls the normal process of genesis and that results in the premature demise of vegetation and lack of proper growth in nature. Liver disease, tremors, fear, contracture or flaccidity of the tendons and bones, and when severe, convulsions can be common. If the yearly primary ruling influence is jueyin/wood then the deficiency is supported and it reverts to a harmonious year. If it encounters yangming/metal as the ruling influence, the wood strength declines further in the control cycle, leading to metal attributes of severe drought of the land and rampant insect infestation mostly occurring in the eastern region. During this time extreme atrophy and immobility of the limbs, abscesses and boils, and intestinal parasites may result. If taiyin/earth is the ruling influence, the earth phase becomes out of control and dominates the year with its attributes of heavy humidity and disease of the digestive system.

"In a fire phase year, a harmonious year is characterized by the balanced fire attributes of bright, warm days and flourishing development in nature. In people the heart, chest, blood vessels, and tongue are the sites of disease.

"An excessive year is characterized by a profusion of fire attributes that may bring extreme, destructively hot weather. Manic and agitated states are common, as well as hysteria, malaria, suppurative lesions, and bleeding. The heart, small and large intestines, pericardium, sanjiao and lungs are usually affected, and so are its corresponding channels. If the ruling influence is taiyang/water then the excess state is neutralized and the year will be harmonious. If the ruling influence is shaoyin/heat or shaoyang/fire the destruction becomes magnified. When the hot environment is so extreme it may invite sudden cold spells, rain, frost, or even hailstorms.

"A deficient year is characterized by a shortage of fire attributes that may bring unstable cool weather. In the summer crops are unable to ripen and insects and animals hibernate early. Heart disease and pain are common as well as confusion, memory loss, disorientation, and sadness. If the ruling influence is shaoyang/fire or shaoyin/heat then the deficiency is supported and it reverts to a harmonious year. If it encounters taiyang/water as the ruling influence, the fire strength declines further, leading to water attributes of prolonged cold spells and thunderstorms occurring mostly in the eastern region. If yangming/metal is the ruling influence, the metal phase becomes unchecked and dominates the year with its attributes of drought and disease of the lungs and intestines.

"In an earth phase year a harmonious year is characterized by the balanced earth elemental attributes of moist weather and fertile nourishment that lead to bursting yields. In people the spleen, muscles, and mouth are the sites of disease.

"An excessive year is characterized by a profusion of earth attributes that may bring heavy fog and mist, frequent rains, and soggy soil that lead to poor harvest. The spleen, stomach, kidneys, and bladder as well as their corresponding channels are frequently affected. Abdominal fullness and distension and muscle weakness are the prevalent symptoms. If the ruling influence is taiyang/water then the winter will be particularly wet and edema will be common.

"A deficient year is characterized by a shortage of earth attributes that may bring lack of timely rainfall, resulting in a meager yield. Disease of the spleen and digestion as well as tumors and edema are typical. If the ruling influence is taiyin/earth then the deficiency is supported and it reverts to a harmonious year. If the ruling influence is jueyin/wood then the earth strength weakens and the result is destructive torrential winds in the central regions spreading out to all directions. During this time diarrhea and dysentery with undigested food may result. If taiyang/water is the ruling influence, the water phase becomes dominant with its attributes of flooding and edema.

"In a metal phase year, a harmonious year is characterized by the balanced metal elemental attributes of a cleansing, dry climate, solidification, and natural decline after reaching the zenith. In people the lungs, chest, nose, and skin are the common sites of disease.

"An excessive year is characterized by a profusion of metal attributes that may bring on drought or an early frost and an end to autumn. Similarly, the rapid onset of trauma and infection to the skin may occur. Disease of the lungs, large intestines, liver, and gallbladder and their corresponding channels as well as cough, dyspnea, orthopnea, and thirst are prevalent. If the ruling influence is shaoyang/fire or shaoyin/heat, then the excess metal will be kept under check. If the ruling influence is taiyang/water the subsequent winter will see severe cold and kidney and bone problems.

"A deficient year is characterized by a shortage of metal attributes that may allow the fire phase to become dominant and manifest severe heat spells that extend well into the autumn. Imbalance causes irritability, impatience, laryngitis, delirium, syncope, cough and asthma, sneezing, and nosebleeds. If the ruling influence is yangming/metal then the deficiency is supported and reverts to a harmonious year. If the ruling influence is shaoyang/fire or shaoyin/heat, the metal is overcome by fire and displays the fire attributes occurring in the western regions that we described earlier. However, immediately following the extreme heat spell will appear severe cold, frost, and hailstorms that usher in the early arrival of winter.

"In a water phase year, a harmonious year is characterized by the balanced water elemental attributes of cold weather, hibernation, and the quiet reservation of the latent life that anticipates its next awakening. In people the kidneys, lower back, knees, and the bones and marrow are the sites of disease.

"An excessive year is characterized by a profusion of water attributes that may induce severe snowstorms and deep freeze that can be quite destructive. Disease of the kidneys, bladder, heart, and small intestine and their corresponding channels as well as chills, joint and back pain, edema, and chest pains can occur during this time. Furthermore, the water humiliates the earth phase in the countercontrol cycle and induces digestive disorders along with rampant mist and persistent rain.

"A deficient year is characterized by a shortage of water attributes that may bring warming trends that extend the growth period of nature; this eventually depletes the underground aquifers. Conditions that arise as a result are constipation, dry stools, atrophy and weakness of the limbs, and lack of clarity. When encountering taiyin/earth as the ruling influence one will see in the northern regions extraordinary wet climate. In the human body this leads to obstruction or difficulty passing urine.

"There, as you can see, the variations of each phase year can bring about tremendous imbalance and suffering to people."

Huang Di asked, "Why does climate differ by region, and do the various regions have a bearing on the human life span?"

Qi Bo replied, "The northern and western regions are generally mountains and high deserts, and therefore tend to be cold and cool, respectively. The southern and eastern regions are generally plains and forests and therefore tend to be hot and warm, respectively. In cooler climates people are more susceptible to external cold and internal heat as well as to edemic and bloating conditions, whereas in warmer climates people suffer more from external heat and internal cold as well as from skin lesions. Incidently, in treatment, a physician should approach cool climate disease with cooling herbals so as to keep the interior from overheating; in warmer climates warming herbals would be more appropriate to keep the yang in the interior. Generally speaking, higher altitudes and colder climates slow the natural process and are conducive for living longer, while the lower plains with a hotter climate hastens the growth and decline process.

Huang Di asked, "Why is it that during some phase years the corresponding organ should be affected but is not?"

Qi Bo replied, "This is because the body is a microcosm that reflects and responds to the changes in the macrocosm. When the ruling atmospheric influence overrules the organs within, the human body will react accordingly. For example, during a year when shaoyang/fire is the primary ruling influence while the jueyin/wind is the secondary influence, one shall observe a severe heat spell in nature in the first half of the year with effects on people that include sneezing, cough, nosebleed, mouth ulcers, edema in the upper body, and chill and fever. One shall observe windstorms in the second half of the year, however, with effects on people that include acute onset of chest and epigastric pain, obstructions, and syncope.

"During a year when yangming/dryness dominates as the primary influence, while the shaoyin/heat is the secondary ruling influence, one will likely see withering droughts and, in people, rib pain, red eyes, dizziness, tremors, atrophy of tendon and ligaments, and inability to stand for any length of time in the first half of the year. In the second half of the year, a severe heat spell disrupts hibernation and the water is unable to freeze, while in people befall heat stroke, scanty dark urination, and malaria along with severe angina.

"During a year when taiyang/cold and taiyin/dampness dominate as the primary and secondary ruling influences, respectively, the first half of the year will see abnormal cold weather that manifests dry retching, sadness, sneezes, uncontrollable yawning, restlessness, forgetfulness, and in extreme cases, angina. In the second half of the year one shall observe a wet climate and people suffering with edema, stomach fullness, anorexia, numbness, stiffness, and abscess lesions.

"During a year when jueyin/wind and shaoyin/heat are the primary and secondary ruling influences, respectively, the first half of the year will tend to be windy and people will suffer with heaviness, vertigo, tinnitus, weak muscles, and anorexia. In the second half of the year patients will likely present acute dysentery with bloody stools. The weather is abnormally hot through the end of the year.

"During a year when shaoyin/heat and yangming/dryness are the primary and secondary influences, respectively, the first half of the year will be characterized by extreme heat spells that cause dyspnea, vomiting, chills and fever, sneezing, nasal obstruction and bleeding, and severe boil conditions in people. The second half of the year will likely see a cool, dry climate that affects people by causing chest pain and persistent sighing.

"During a year when taiyin/dampness and taiyang/coldness are the primary and secondary influences, respectively, the first half of the year will tend to wetness with people suffering from fullness in the chest and abdomen, infertility, impotence, back pain, stiffness, and syncope. The second half of the year will likely see an early winter freeze that in people causes abdominal pain, anorexia, dysuria, and a salty taste in the mouth. It is the various energetic circuits and cycles that act as checks and balances in the entire ecosystem that give rise to aberration as well as consistencies in nature."

Huang Di asked, "How does one go about rectifying these various imbalances?"

Qi Bo replied, "When treating a deficient condition arising from deficiency of the circuit or influence, one should administer herbals that correspond to the deficient elemental phase. In contrast, an excess condition deserves to be treated with herbals that correspond to an elemental phase that checks the excess element in the five elemental control cycle. For instance, a wood deficient condition should be treated with sour, warming, and green herbals. A wood excess condition should be treated with pungent, cooling, and white herbals. When treating febrile disease, administer a cooling herbal decoction while warm. Similarly for cold conditions administer a warming herbal decoction cold."

Huang Di asked, "How do you care for someone with a mass that appears and disappears without reason?"

Qi Bo replied, "If there is not a fixed mass then one should approach by determining the strength of the person and the pathogen. If it is deficient, fortify immediately. If it is accompanied by an external pathogen then dispel it first before nourishing the weakness with dietetics. In this way, once the blood and qi are balanced, the condition will vanish."

Huang Di asked, "Are there any rules regarding administering herbal medicine?"

Qi Bo replied, "Specifically, when administering medicine, once the health is sixty percent recovered, withdraw the extreme toxic herbal; once the health is seventy percent recovered, withdraw the moderate toxic herbal; once the health is eighty percent recovered, withdraw the mildly toxic herbal; once the health is ninety percent recovered, withdraw the nontoxic herbal. Follow up with special food herbs and dietetic remedies for regeneration. Following this principle, a physician will be successful in patients' care.

Huang Di asked, "How does one go about maintaining absolute health and well-being?"

Qi Bo replied, "Health and well-being can be achieved only by remaining centered with one's spirit, guarding against squandering one's energy, maintaining the constant flow of one's qi and blood, adapting to the changing seasonal and yearly macrocosmic influences, and nourishing one's self preventively."

Huang Di gratefully thanked Qi Bo for imparting his wisdom.

CHAPTER 71

—

THE SIX MACROCOSMIC
INFLUENCES

—

HUANG DI commented, "I would like to hear further details on each of the various circuit years, its ruling influences, and its excess, harmonious, and deficient states."

Qi Bo replied, "First of all one needs to determine the elemental phase, the yearly and seasonal primary and secondary ruling atmospheric influences of the circuit year. Then ascertain the excess or deficient nature of the ruling influence in relation to the various cycles of the five elemental phase law. Once this information is secured, one will be able to estimate the meteorological and epidemiological tendencies of the year. Utilize herbs that would counteract the effects of the pathogenic influences. Restrain the excess while fortifying the deficient. Take preventive measures by living a healthy, balanced life and consume appropriate foods corresponding to the seasonal needs.

"For example, for the years that contain chen or xu as branches, the corresponding primary ruling influence is always taiyang/cold and the secondary ruling influence is taiyin/damp. Generally the years tend to be cold and damp, and therefore treatment should utilize bitter and warming herbals to dry and dispel cold. When the years ruled by taiyang/cold concur with the wood phase stem ren, harmony is characterized by a gentle wind, while a destructive windstorm indicates an excess state. Dizziness, vertigo, photophobia, and blurry vision are common symptoms of illness. When taiyang/cold years concur with the fire phase stem wu, harmony is characterized by normal summer heat while extreme heat indicates an excess state. Restless and febrile disease are common. When taiyang/cold years concur with the earth phase stem jia, harmony is characterized by an appropriate amount of rainfall and humidity while heavy thunderstorms that lead to flooding indicate an excess state. When taiyang/cold years concur with the metal phase stem gen, harmony is characterized by a cooling and drying trend while premature decay of nature indicates an excess state. When taiyang/cold years concur with the water phase stem bing, harmony is characterized by a normal cold and freezing climate while heavy hail and snowstorms indicate an excess state.

"Seasonally, each of the six step periods will reflect specific character-istics of the atmospheric influence. During taiyang/cold years, the first step will exhibit febrile disease of epidemic nature accompanied by fever, head-ache, vomiting, and skin infections. The second step will exhibit chest and abdominal fullness and distension because of the stagnation of yang. The third step will exhibit carbuncle, dysentery, disorientation, and restlessness. The fourth step will exhibit febrile disease accompanied by muscle weak-ness and bloody dysentery. The fifth step will exhibit normal unaffected health. The last step will exhibit miscarriage in women.

"During years ruled by the yangming/dryness influence, the branches always correspond to mao or you and the secondary ruling influence is always shaoyin/heat. Generally yangming years are cool and dry in the first half and extremely hot in the second half. Therefore treatment should uti-lize salty, bitter, and pungent herbals to lubricate the dryness and clear the heat. Diaphoretic, clearing, and dispersing methods should be employed. When yangming/dry years concur with the wood phase stem ding, the impacts of the wood phase is ameliorated by the yangming or metal phase, its controller. When yangming/dry years concur with the fire phase stem kui, the impact of the fire phase is subdued owing to its deficient state that would cause it to be impotent in controlling the yangming/dry influence. When yangming/dry years concur with the earth phase stem si, the yang-ming/influence is in a dominant position in the control cycle; thus no effect from the earth phase is realized. When yangming/dry years concur with the metal phase stem yi, the effects of the yangming/influence is mag-nified because the great circuit stem, the atmospheric influence, and the branch all correspond to metal. These are referred to as tai yi tian fu years. When yangming/dry years concur with the water phase stem xin, the cir-cuit impact is minimized because of its nonthreatening position in the five elemental cycle.

"Seasonally, the first step during the yangming/dry years will tend to display fever, nasal discharge and bleeding, sneezing, vomit, hypersomnia, edema in the face, abdominal distension, and dysuria. The second step will display sudden death from epidemic infections. The third step will display conditions of alternating chills and fever. The fourth step will display short-ness of breath, thirst, chest pain, blood in the stools, arthralgia, shaking, delirium, abscesses and boils, fainting, and malaria. The fifth step will dis-play generally good health. The last step will display febrile diseases.

"During the years ruled by the shaoyang/fire influence, the corre-sponding branches are always yin or shen. Its secondary influence is invari-ably jueyin/wind. Gererally shaoyang/fire years tend to be hot in the first part and windy in the latter part of the year. People are susceptible to conditions of fever and chills, diarrhea, deafness, vomit, eye infections, skin lesions, abdominal distension, edema, and malaria. Treatment should utilize salty, pungent, and sour herbals to cool the fire and disperse the wind. Clearing, diuretic, lubricating, and dispersing methods should be em-ployed. When shaoyang/fire years concur with the wood phase stem ren, imbalance tends to cause dizziness, vertigo, hypochondria, neuralgia, and anxiety. When shaoyang/fire years concur with the fire phase stem wu, imbalance tends to cause chest pain, bleeding, and heat in the upper body and head area. When shaoyang/fire years concur with the earth phase stem jia, imbalance tends to cause heavy limbs, edema, and mucous congestion. When shaoyang/fire years concur with the metal phase stem gen, imbal-ance tends to cause problems involving the shoulder and the back. When shaoyang/fire years concur with the water phase stem bing, imbalance tends to give rise to cold conditions and swelling.

"Seasonally the first step during shaoyang/fire years will manifest cough, asthma, skin lesions, rib pain, abnormal uterine bleeding, and blood stagnation in the upper body, causing broken capillaries in the eyes and headache. The second step will manifest heat stagnation in the upper body causing fever, headache, disorientation, suppurative skin lesions, throat and chest discomfort, cough, and vomit. The third step will manifest fever, deafness, infection and bleeding in the eyes, nosebleed, sneezing, controlla-ble yawning, and throat pain, and in severe cases sudden death may befall. The fourth step will manifest heavy limbs and abdominal swelling. The fifth step will manifest a generally colder than usual climate. At this time people are encouraged to stay indoors and protect themselves from the elements. The last step will manifest cough, chest pain, and incontinence of both urine and bowels.

"For the years that are ruled by taiyin/damp the corresponding branches are always chou or wei and its secondary ruling influence is always taiyang/cold. Generally the year is characterized by heavy rainfall in the first half and darker, colder days in the last half of the year. Treatment should include aromatic, bitter, and warming herbals to dry the dampness and dispel the coldness. During these years people tend to suffer from conditions of abdominal swelling, edema, extreme coldness of the limbs, and muscle spasms. During excess circuit years, farmers should delay planting their crops in higher ground and during deficient years the reverse should be followed. When taiyin/damp years concur with the wood phase stem ding, the circuit phase is deficient and therefore it has minimal impact to the year. When taiyin/damp years concur with the fire phase stem kui, the circuit phase is also deficient and unable to fuel the power of the influence. Therefore it is also a minor factor. When taiyin/damp years concur with the earth phase stem si, the circuit year is also deficient and therefore does not make much impact. When taiyin/damp years concur with the metal phase stem yi, the circuit year is deficient and again does not have an effect. Last, when taiyin/damp years concur with the water phase xin, the same thing is also true and thus it does not become a factor in affecting the outcome of weather and disease.

"Seasonally, the first step during taiyin/damp years will typically present with stiff and painful joints, heaviness, and lethargy; the second step with plague; the third step with cold and damp conditions of edema, chest and abdominal distension, and heaviness; the fourth step with fever, abdominal swelling, feverish sensation in the chest, edema, sudden bleeding, and malaria; the fifth step with conditions in the superficial level; and the last step with severe chills and arthralgia in the spine and the joints.

"During the years ruled by shaoyin/heat and yangming/dry as the primary and secondary ruling influences, respectively, the corresponding branches are always zi or wu. Generally the weather is hotter interspersed with rainstorms in the first half and cooler weather in the second half of the year. People typically suffer from cough, red, swollen, and painful eyes, bleeding, pain in the chest and lower back, abdominal fullness, edema in the upper body, and throat dryness. Treatment should include salty and cold herbals to clear heat and lubricate dryness. In severe cases bitter and sour herbals may be employed to purge the heat the rehydrate the dryness. When shaoyin/heat years concur with the wood phase stem ren, imbalance will present rib pains. When shaoyin/heat years concur with the fire phase stem wu, imbalance will present heat stagnation in the head, leading to bleeding. When shaoyin/heat years concur with the earth phase stem jia, imbalance will present epigastric fullness and heaviness in the body. When shaoyin/heat years concur with the metal phase stem gen, imbalance will present diarrhea with clear discharge. When shaoyin/heat years concur with the water phase stem bing, imbalance will present severe chills in the lower limbs.

"Seasonally during shaoyin/heat years, the first step will typically display pain and contracture in the spine and joints; the second step will display conditions of dysuria, qi stagnation in the head region, and eye disease; the third step will display chest pain, alternating fever and chills, cough, red eyes, and syncope; the fourth step will display fever and chills, dry throat, jaundice, nosebleed, and edema; the fifth step will display generally good health; and the last step will display diarrhea and conditions on the superficial level and the rib area.

"During the years where jueyin/wind and shaoyang/fire are the primary and secondary ruling influences, respectively, the branches are always ji or hai. Generally, the years are characterized by windy weather in the first half and unusually warm weather in the last half of the year. People tend to suffer from heat conditions in the lower and wind conditions in the upper body. Treatment should consist of pungent herbals to disperse the wind from the upper body and salty herbals to purge the heat from the lower body. Since all the five phase stems that are combined with ji and hai indicate deficient states, the impact from circuit year energetics is very minimal. The jueyin/wind years will be mainly dominated by their atmospheric influences.

"Seasonally during jueyin/wind years, the first step will typically display conditions involving the right, lower parts of the body; the second step will display conditions involving the middle regions of the body; the third step will display dizziness, vertigo, tinnitus, tremors, and excess tears; the fourth step will display jaundice, edema, and conditions involving the left, upper body; the fifth step will display superficial conditions; and the final step will display generally good health."

Huang Di asked, "Thank you for your exhaustive explanation of the different years dominated by the atmospheric influences as they encounter the impacts of the sixty-year circuit. What would happen, however, if the meteorological manifestations do not match that of the great circuit phase?"

Qi Bo replied, "If the correct weather does not manifest at the beginning of a circuit year it is called deficiency. If it manifests before the start of the circuit year it is called excess. If it manifests just on time, this is normal.

Anytime when there is imbalance in nature, catastrophes will descend upon the land and its people."

Huang Di asked, "What causes natural catastrophes to occur?"

Qi Bo replied, "In the five elemental phase energetics, the control cycle keeps each of the elemental phases in check and thus maintains order and harmony. However, in nature the controlled elemental phase when restrained to the extreme will rebel, and the result is often dramatic and devastating. Take the example of a dominant wood phase that controls the earth phase, which in the extreme will generate lightning storms and calamitous flash floods. Similarly, people will display conditions of vomiting, abdominal rumbling, and dysentery with the same acute onset and urgency that mimic the phenomena of nature.

Huang Di asked, "How does one go about addressing conditions arising from rebellious macrocosmic influences?"

Qi Bo replied, "When the wood phase is rebellious, seek to disperse and circulate the stagnant liver energy. When the fire phase is rebellious, seek to clear and cool the heat from the heart. When the earth phase is rebellious, seek to purge, cast up, and shift the obstruction in the spleen and the digestion. When the metal phase is rebellious, seek to ventilate the lung energy. And finally when the water phase is rebellious, seek to reduce the water retention from the kidneys by diuretic methods."

Huang Di asked, "What are the general rules governing the use of herbal medicine?"

Qi Bo replied, "When heat predominates the environment, avoid warming and hot herbs and when cold predominates the environment stay away from cooling and cold herbs. When this rule is violated, the sick will deteriorate and the healthy will become ill."

Huang Di asked, "What are the manifestations of this violation?"

Qi Bo replied, "When cold is aggravated the patient will suffer from chills, abdominal swelling and hardness, severe pain, and diarrhea whereas heat will cause fever; vomit; skin infections; restlessness; dysentery; convulsions; bleeding from the nose, mouth, and the bowels; pain in the head, joints, and muscles; obstruction of the urine; and bowels."

Huang Di asked, "Are there exceptions to this rule?"

Qi Bo replied, "Yes. The exception to this rule is when the need arises to promote diaphoresis in order to expel the pathogen from the exterior. In this situation one can use hot herbs regardless of the seasonal factor. Similarly, when the case calls for purging of pathogens from the interior, cold herbs can be employed notwithstanding."

Huang Di asked, "What about the use of herbal medicine for each of the sixty circuit years? Are there general rules to follow?"

Qi Bo replied, "Yes. A physician will dispense care and the use of herbals depending upon the cause of the illness. Within each year there are three macrocosmic pathogenic factors to consider. The elemental phase of the circuit is the first, the primary atmospheric ruling influence is the second, and the secondary ruling influence is the third of the factors that can all interact and become harmful to living organisms. A dominant factor that is the cause of illness should be addressed with proper herbal treatment. For instance, during the jia/zi and jia/wu years the great circuit is the earth phase, the primary ruling influence is shaoyin/heat, and the secondary ruling influence is yangming/dry. If the earth phase is excess and dominates, administer bitter and warming herbs to dry up the damp tendencies. Similarly if the shaoyin/heat is dominant, use salty and cold herbs to cool the heat; and if the yangming/dry is dominant, treat with sour and warming herbs. This principle applies to any given year within the sixty-year cycle."

Huang Di asked, "In pregnant women are there any dangers in taking potent herbs?"

Qi Bo replied, "No harm will be done when the condition calls for such action."

Huang Di commented, "This knowledge passed down from the ancient achieved beings embodies the highest wisdom of the universe. I will treasure it in the sacred archives and I shall not even touch its pages until I have fasted and cleansed myself for seven days. I will also exercise the utmost prudence in passing on this knowledge only to the virtuous."

CHAPTER 72

—

ACUPUNCTURE
IN EPIDEMIOLOGY

—

HUANG DI asked, "As extremes and disharmonies occur during the interplay of the natural elements, plagues and disease arise to cause sufferings in people. What are the ways that can help to prevent the effects of imbalance from the macrocosm upon human beings?"

Qi Bo replied, "You have asked a question that deserves an answer in depth. Generally a physician needs to be versed in the laws of the universe and its interactive dynamics, and to have a firm grasp of the knowledge of acupuncture, in order to know when to fortify a deficient and when to reduce an excessive state and how to maintain constancy of energy flow in patients. There are several factors that throw the normal weather patterns off its track.

"For example, when an atmospheric influence is repressed by the current primary ruling atmospheric influence in the preset sequence, an extreme catastrophe and subsequent epidemics will often follow during its sequentially occurring circuit year. Acupuncture can be applied as a preventive measure against epidemic infection. In the human body located on each channel are a set of points identified with each of the five elements. On the yang channels they are represented by jing/well-metal, rong/spring-water, shu/stream-wood, jing/river-fire, and he/sea-earth. On the yin channels they are represented by jing/well-wood, rong/spring-fire, shu/stream-earth, jing/river-metal, and he/sea-water. By acupuncturing the corresponding elemental point of the organ system that is the most susceptible, that organ system will become balanced and thus avert any potential disorder.

"More specifically, when jueyin/wood is repressed by a primary ruling influence of yangming/metal in the five elemental control cycle, some form of natural meteorological disasters may occur when its ruling circuit year arrives. Consequently, people will be very ill and subject to epidemics. For prevention of potential ills a physician should acupuncture his subjects on the jing/well-wood point of the foot jueyin/liver channel. Similarly, acupuncture the rong/spring-fire point of the hand jueyin/pericardium channel for shaoyin/fire repression by taiyang/water; acupuncture the shu/stream-earth point of the foot taiyin/spleen channel for taiyin/earth repression by jueyin/wood; acupuncture the jing/river-metal point of the hand taiyin/lung channel for yangming/metal repression by shaoyang/fire; acupuncture the he/sea-water point of the foot shaoyin/kidney channel for taiyang/water repression by taiyin/earth.

"Additionally, when an atmospheric influence is repressed by the current secondary ruling influence in the preset sequence, an extreme catastrophe and consequent epidemics will also follow during its sequentially occurring circuit year. In this case, acupuncture the aggressor phase channel to tonify the elemental point of the repressed on the yin channel, and the elemental point that is the controller of the aggressor influence.

"For example, when the jueyin/wood influence is repressed by the secondary ruling influence of yangming/metal, acupuncture the jing/well-wood point on the hand taiying/lung-metal channel and the he/sea-earth point on the hand yangming/large intestine-metal channel. The same formula applies to all other channels similar to this scenario.

"Furthermore, when the ruling influence of the current year is bu quan zheng—does not appear on time, owing to the excess of the prior year's influence, that is, the prior year's influence continues to exert its meteorologic characteristics—conflict will occur between the current year's ruling and the prior year's ruling influences, leading to inevitable catastrophes. In this case, acupuncture the rong/spring point on the corresponding channel of the current year's ruling influence. For example, when jueyin/wood of the current year does not appear on time, owing to taiyang/water of the prior year not departing on time, the delayed onset of jueyin/wood will lead to certain devastations. As a preventive measure, acupuncture the rong/spring-fire point on the foot jueyin/liver channel to strengthen the control phase of fire over water. The same formula should be used in other situations involvling a similar scenario.

"Finally, when the prior year's secondary ruling influence is so excess that it is bu tui wei—refuses to depart on time—in the current year it can also exert unnatural impact to the environment. In this case, acupuncture the he/sea points on its corresponding channels. For example, when a given year comes to an end and the secondary ruling influence, say, jueyin/ wood, does not depart on time and continues to dominate into the next year, acupuncture the he/sea-water point to weaken the source of the jueyin in the creative cycle of the five elemental phases. Repeat this guideline to other situations of similar scenario.

"Successful application of these acupuncture guidelines will prevent the parallel energy disorder within individual human beings and will lessen the coming epidemiological impacts of a perverse atmospheric influence."

Huang Di asked, "During a given year if the ruling influences either do not take their place or depart on time, natural catastrophes and epidemics may follow as a result. What other preventive or treatment methods can be employed to help avert or lessen the negative impacts?"

Qi Bo replied, "When the ruling influences are off track one year, about three years later an epidemic will be certain to strike. Perform acupuncture on the shu/stream points of the dominant phase channel and the phase channel to which it exerts direct control. This will prepare the body and prevent disorders from fermenting.

"For instance, if the ruling influences are off track during the jia/zi year and the seasons do not manifest as they should, in about three years an epidemic will strike that is dominant in earth/damp characteristics. In this case acupuncture the shu/stream point of the kidney channel and the spleen channel to sedate against the impending dominant earth energy. Subsequent to the treatment, the patient should avoid being away from home, especially at night-time, and should remain serene and consume only a vegetarian diet for seven days. Each morning at the hours of yin/3-5 A.M. one should face south and swallow the heavenly energy seven times while deeply inhaling to strengthen one's zheng/antipathogenic qi. Apply this principle in other comparably occurring years."

Huang Di asked, "The epidemic infections are often deadly and contagious. Are there any ways that health workers can prevent being infected?"

Qi Bo replied, "People with strong zheng/antipathogenic qi do not succumb to epidemic infections. Let me share with you some of the ways. Before entering a medical facility a health worker must focus the mind and summon the indefeatable antipathogenic forces to protect the body against any possible invasion. This worker should practice visualizing a strong liver with green energy emanating from it to the east and producing vibrant vegetation; a white energy emanating from robust lungs to the west turning into metal armor and weapons; a red energy emanating from an active heart to the south creating radiant light; a deep blue energy emanating from solid kidneys to the north forming a formidable sea; and a yellow energy emanating from a sturdy spleen in the middle manifesting the substantial earth. Further, the worker should always see in the mind the glistening rays of the north star on the vertex of the head. Several other methods involve Dao-in and Qi Gong practices at sunrise on the first day of spring, bathing with special herbs after the second solar term of rain water, and taking herbs containing realgar and cinnabar made with exclusive methods for ten days prior to the onset of any epidemic. With these practices and methods, this worker will be safe to contact pathogens without becoming ill."

Huang Di asked, "I would like to know how to remedy a situation where the patient was already predisposed to illness because of weakness in a particular organ system, and encounters a corresponding pathogen that specifically attacks the organ and causes the person's shen/spirit to be disturbed as well."

Qi Bo replied, "A person becomes ill from being attacked by a pathogen. If that person happens to be susceptible because of preexisting organ deficiency while encountering an excessive pathogenic atmospheric influence, that person will surely succumb to illness and death as the shen/spirit collapses. For example, a person with liver/wood weakness and an unsettled hun/liver spirit encounters a year when the ruling influence of jueyin/wind-wood is deficient as well, which makes it a triple weakness. Under this circumstance, syncope and death are certain. However, if the body remains warm, one can resuscitate by acupuncturing the patient's yuan/source point on the gallbladder channel and the shu/stream point on the liver channel. The same treatment method applies to all other triple weakness conditions."

Huang Di asked, "If a single organ is diseased, would it not affect the rest of the body and cause disorder of other organs?"

Qi Bo replied, "You are keen in your observation. Indeed, the entire body functions as a single entity, much like a kingdom where from the emperor down to the manager of the warehouse, each has a job to fulfill in order to make the state prosperous. The human body is no different, and treatment of disease must take into account the whole body so as to propitiously address all the related problems. Ultimately, by following the Tao and implementing its life-enhancing maxims, one can expect to live harmoniously in wellness with the ever-changing universe."

CHAPTER 73

—

ETIOLOGY OF DISEASE

—

HUANG DI asked, "What circumstances constitute a lapse in the cyclical intercourse between the heavenly and the earthly energies?"

Qi Bo replied, "What you asked is in reference to the primary and the secondary ruling influences that appear in a preset sequential way. When the atmospheric influences from heaven appear as they should at the correct yearly and seasonal interval, there is harmony. A lapse occurs when the influences are off track: that is, they either do not depart on time or appear on time; the result is then instability in nature and disease in human beings."

Huang Di inquired, "Can you elaborate on the mechanism behind these lapses?"

Qi Bo responded, "The primary ruling influence represents the influential heavenly energy that dictates the meteorologic trends of the first half of a year, while the secondary ruling influence represents the native earthly energy that dictates the last half of a year. When the secondary ruling influence is excess, it could inhibit the arrival of the succeeding primary ruling influence. Further, when the yearly elemental phase circuit is excess, it could also dominate the current year's ruling influences. The interference of the normal cycles will result in differing degrees of damage, depending on the cause."

Huang Di asked, "Tell me more about the five-elemental-phase dynamics within the energetic cycles."

Qi Bo replied, "The different cosmic energies all function within the five-elemental-phase paradigm. In the creative cycle the characteristics of an elemental phase is accentuated, while in the destructive or control cycle a decrease is observed.

"For instance, during chen and xu branch years, because of the prior year's excess metal, the jueyin/wood seasonal influence becomes repressed by the metal and is unable to exert its normal influence during the first step of the year in the spring. A similar scenario occurs during gen/xu years when the gen stem is the excess yang metal stem; hence, the metal element dominates the circuit, which then represses the jueyin/wood seasonal influence.

"During these years when wood is repressed by metal, in spring, nature will display cooling and destructive trends of autumn/metal. Spring will bring frosts that stunt the beginning growth of all things and cause people to suffer from dry, sore throat, edema in the limbs, and joint pains. When wood is repressed to the extreme, great windstorms will arise, destroying everything in its path. People will fall victim to stroke and paralysis.

"Another sistuation with the same results is played out during chou and wei branch years when the former excess ruling influence of shaoyin/heat refuses to depart on time and the current year's phase circuit happens to be metal. The jueyin/wood influence cannot exert its normal seasonal influence because of repression by metal; therefore, autumnal characteristics will appear in spring."

Huang Di said, "I would like to hear about what happens when a ruling influence does not appear or depart on time."

Qi Bo replied, "When the characteristics of the former year's ruling influence remains after the first day of the current year, it prevents the succeding current year's ruling influence from taking its place.

"For instance, when jueyin/wood cannot take its place and appear on time, one sees withering of vegetation instead of genesis. People will most likely complain of eye disease, tendon and ligament sprains, anger fits, and disease of the urinary tract.

"When the ruling influence of a given year is excess and continues to dominate well into the following year, this is called 'the ruling influence does not depart on time.'

"For instance, when jueyin/wood does not depart on time, one will see in nature great winds but no rain, and thus vegetation will fail to germinate in the spring. People will suffer from febrile disease, joint pain, headache, eye pain, restlessness, dry, sore throat, and paralysis."

Huang Di asked, "Can you generalize about the energetic tendencies within the sixty-year cycle?"

Qi Bo replied, "In the sixty-year cycle there are thirty yang years alternating with thirty yin years. The yang years are excess circuit years, except for six of the thirty years where the succeeding ruling influences cannot appear on time and which are therefore considered deficient years."

Huang Di asked, "What is the mechanism behind sudden death in disease?"

Qi Bo replied, "When a person who is deficient in qi of a particular viscera and who engages in emotional activities that further dissipate the spirit of that viscera encounters a given year in which the corresponding ruling influence is also deficient, it is referred to as 'triple jeopardy' and results in sudden death.

"For instance, suppose a person suffering from heart qi deficiency during a year ruled by a deficient shaoyin/heat atmospheric influence becomes startled and overly stimulated by emotional trauma that dissipates his shen/spirit. Sudden death may ensue when his shen collapses. This is the result of triple jeopardy.

"Therefore, when the qi and shen are present and sound, no pathogen can invade a person, even when the cycles of nature are disruptive and plagues are near."

CHAPTER 74

—

ESSENTIALS OF DISEASE
AND THERAPY

—

HUANG DI stated, "People and nature are inseparable. In nature the cyclical movement of the heavenly bodies produces atmospheric influences that exert control over the rhythms of the seasons and is responsible for change to the myriad living and nonliving things. These cycles are repeated endlessly with patterns of predictability, and yet simultaneously with a tendency toward chaos. It is this chaos in the macrocosm that upsets the balance of the delicate ecology within people that produces disease."

Huang Di then asked, "Please tell me what are the essentials of disease and therapy."

Qi Bo replied, "The six atmospheric influences of jueyin/wind, shaoyin/heat, taiyin/damp, shaoyang/fire, yangming/dryness, and taiyang/cold that occur in nature form the basis for the birth and death of all things as well as for illnesses in people. Each influence is dominant, or rules normally in a sequential way on a seasonal and yearly rotation. It is within this rotation that chaos may occur, when a guest influence comes to dominate at inappropriate times, that the balanced ecology becomes disturbed. To restore balance within people one may utilize herbal medicine that possess counter properties to the offending pathogenic influence. For instance if shaoyang/fire was the invading influence, use salty, bitter, and cold herbs to cool and clear the fire. This approach of counteracting the pathogen by using herbs with control properties is called zheng zhu, diametric treatment. Sometimes when the cause of a condition is in opposite nature to the manifested signs and symptoms, for instance, taiyang/cold invasion manifesting fevers, the use of herbs with properties that may be alike to the manifestations such as sweet, pungent, and hot would be called for. In this situation, the approach of using like properties to cure a like manifested condition is called fan zhi, homeopathic treatment."

Huang Di asked, "How do the pulses reflect these differing yearly circuits?"

Qi Bo replied, "If one's pulses do not correspond to the prevailing influence, that indicates trouble. The normal pulses should be slightly wiry for jueyin, flooding for shaoyin, sinking for taiyin, large and floating for shaoyang, short and choppy for yangming, and large and long for taiyang. If the influence is present and the pulses are absent, or if the influence has passed but the pulses are still present, or any other variant from the normal are considered pathological."

Huang Di inquired, "Can you please describe the pathology for each organ system and its connection with the atmospheric influences?"

Qi Bo responded, "Symptoms of tremors and shaking of the limbs, dizziness, and vertigo are usually caused by wind and associated with the liver. Many conditions of contraction and spasms are usually due to cold and associated with the kidneys. Symptoms of rapid, labored breathing, chest tightness, and obstruction are caused by dryness and related to the lungs. Symptoms of edema, bloating, and distension are usually caused by dampness and associated with the spleen. Symptoms of disorientation, confusion, convulsions and seizures, pain, and itching are usually due to fire and related to the heart. Symptoms of either obstruction or incontinence of urine and feces and many types of syncope are usually due to disorder of the lower jiao/cavity. Symptoms of nausea, vomit, cough, asthma, and many types of wei/flaccidity conditions are usually due to disorder of the upper and middle jiao. Symptoms of neck and jaw stiffness and spasm and contracture of muscles and tendons are usually due to dampness. Symptoms of lockjaw, mental and emotional disturbance, anxiety, and swelling and inflammation are usually due to fire. Many acute-onset conditions with generalized stiffness are usually caused by wind. Symptoms of abdominal swelling, borborygmus, tympany of the abdominal cavity, vomit of foul matter, and acute dysentery of blood and mucus in the stools are usually due to heat. Symptoms of chills and diarrhea with clear and watery stools are usually caused by cold. When caring for a patient, a physician discovers the cause and understands the pathology, analyzes the zang and fu organ connections, counteracts the pathogens, revives the flow of qi and blood, and finally restores the balance of the human body."

Huang Di asked, "Can you discuss the nature and property of different herbs by their flavors and the composition of an effective formula?"

Qi Bo replied, "Pungent and sweet herbs disperse and fortify. Bland herbs promote diuresis and get rid of dampness. These herbs are considered yang. Sour and bitter herbs induce expelling in either direction. Salty herbs lubricate and dissolve hardening. These herbs are considered yin.

"The composition of a herbal formula is dependent on several criteria. First determine the seriousness of the patient's condition. Second find out the nature of the pathogen or deficiency. Third ascertain the treatment principle. There are three proportionally different formulas. A large formula is used for severe and complex conditions and involves one king herb, three ministerial herbs and nine assistant herbs. A medium formula is used for moderately complex situations and consists of one king herb, three ministerial herbs and five assistant herbs. A small formula is used for relatively mild cases and is made up of one king herb and two ministerial herbs. Treatment principles consist of warming to dispel cold, cooling to clear heat, dispersing to remove congestion, purging to eliminate buildup, catharsis to dispel water, lubricating to moisten dryness, fortifying to strengthen deficiency, decelerating to arrest acute progression, invigorating to accelerate flow, inducing vomiting to expel food or phlegm, calming to tranquilize anxiety, and softening to dissolve mass. Other methods such as bathing with herbs and massage can be used as adjunctive therapies."

Huang Di asked, "Can you please tell me about the disease of each of the primary ruling influences and its corresponding therapy?"

Qi Bo replied, "Yes, allow me to summarize it for you. During years ruled by jueyin/wind people tend to suffer distress to the spleen and stomach because the wood phase overacts on the earth phase. Symptoms include pain and discomfort of the stomach and ribs, obstructed sensation in the throat, tongue stiffness, bulimia, diarrhea, dysuria, and ascites. To assist in the recovery one should dispense pungent and cooling herbs as the king constituent of an herbal formula to disperse the wind; bitter and sweet herbs as the minister to strengthen the spleen; sour herbs as assistant to mollify the liver; and sweet herbs as diplomat to retard the swiftness of the disease. The absence of the pulse of the dorsal artery of the feet near the chongyang (ST42) point indicates collapse of the stomach qi and inevitable death.

"During the years ruled by shaoyin/heat people tend to suffer problems of their lungs and large intestines because the fire phase overacts on the metal phase. Symptoms include chest tightness and agitation, cough, blood in the mucus, dyspnea, asthma, retch, vomit, abdominal distension, bloody diarrhea, dark urine, and suppurative skin lesions. One should employ salty and cold herbs as the king; bitter and sweet herbs as the minister; and sour herbs as the assistant constituent of a prescription. The absence of a pulse of the radial artery near the chize (LU5) point indicates imminent death.

"During the years rules by taiyin/damp people tend to suffer trouble of their kidneys and bladder because the earth phase overacts on the water phase. Symptoms include pain and stiffness in all the bones and joints of the body, edema, dizziness, vertigo, anorexia, shortness of breath, difficulty with defecation, anxiety, and fright. One should dispense bitter and hot herbs as king; sour and pungent herbs as minister; bitter herbs as assistant; and bland herbs as diplomat in a herbal formulation. The absence of a pulse of the tibial artery near taixi (K3) indicates a poor prognosis.

"During the years ruled by shaoyang/fire people tend to suffer distress of their lungs and large intestines because the fire phase overacts on the metal phase. Symptoms include headaches, fever, chills, malaria, superficial neuralgia of the skin, edema of the face, difficulty gasping for air, cough, blood in the mucus, chest tightness, agitation, nosebleed, abdominal distension and bloody dysentery. One should dispense sour and cold herbs as king; bitter and sweet herbs as minister; sour herbs as assistant; and bitter herbs as diplomat in a formula. The absence of a pulse of the brachial artery near tianfu (LU3) indicates impending death.

"During the years ruled by yangming/dryness people tend to suffer illness of the liver and gallbladder because the metal phase overacts on the wood phase. Symptoms include pain under the right ribs, malaria, contracture of tendons and ligaments, hernia, blurry vision, eye infections, boils, pelvic pain in females, borborygmus, and diarrhea. One should dispense bitter and warm herbs as king; sour and pungent herbs as minister; and bitter herbs as assistant in an herbal prescription. The absence of a pulse of the dorsal metatarsal artery near taichong (LIV3) indicates imminent death.

"During the years ruled by taiyang/cold people tend to suffer distress of the heart and small intestine because the water phase overacts on the fire phase. Symptoms include angina, palpitation, chest and epigastrium discomfort, thirst, burping, syncope, vomiting of blood, blood in the stool, nosebleed, grief, dizziness and loss of equilibrium, abdominal distension, and fullness. One should dispense pungent and hot herbs as king; sweet and bitter herbs as minister; and salty herbs as assistant in an herbal prescription. The absence of a pulse of the ulnar artery near shenmen (H7) indicates a grave outcome."

Huang Di asked, "Can you please tell me about the disease of each secondary ruling influence and its corresponding therapy?"

Qi Bo replied, "Yes. During the latter half of the years ruled by the secondary ruling influence of jueyin/wind, people tend to suffer from shivers from chills, chest tightness, discomfort of the ribs, bulimia, throat obstruction, abdominal bloating relieved by flatulence, and burping and heaviness of body. Medicate with pungent and cooling herbs as king; bitter herbs as minister; and pungent and sweet herbs as assistant.

"Shaoyin/heat years are prevalent with conditions of alternating chills and fever, skin neuralgia, chest and abdominal discomfort and pain, dyspnea, photophobia, and toothache. Medicate with salty and cold herbs as king; sweet and bitter herbs as minister; and sour and bitter herbs as assistant.

"Taiyin/damp years are rampant with problems of water retention, epigastric pain, deafness, headache, blurry vision, muddled senses, laryngitis, abdominal pain, dysuria, and pain and immobility in the neck, lower back, and hips, calf pain, and tightness of the heel. Medicate with bitter and hot herbs as king; sour and bland herbs as minister; and bitter and bland herbs as assistant.

"Shaoyang/fire years bring about suffering of severe, acute dysentery with abdominal pain, and blood in the stools and urine. Medicate with salty and cold herbs as king; bitter and pungent herbs as minister; and sour and bitter herbs as assistant.

"Yangming/dryness year conditions that are widespread include chest and rib pain with limited mobility of the trunk, vomiting of bitter fluid or retching, feverish on the outer feet, and severe dry skin throughout. Medicate with bitter and warming herbs as king; sweet and pungent herbs as minister; and bitter herbs as assistant.

"Taiyang/cold years are prevalent with conditions of pain in the lower abdomen radiating to the scrotum and lower back, chest pain, and sore throat. Medicate with sweet and hot herbs as king; bitter and pungent herbs as minister; and salty and pungent herbs as assistant."

Huang Di asked, "What if the primary ruling influence does not appear on time and is overruled by another influence—what treatment do you recommend?"

Qi Bo replied, "If jueyin/wind is overruled by yangming/dryness, then medicate with sour and warming herbs as king and sweet and bitter herbs as minister. If shaoyin/heat is overruled by taiyang/cold, then medicate with sweet and warming herbs as king and bitter, sour, and pungent herbs as minister. If taiyin/damp is overruled by shaoyin/heat, then medicate with bitter and cold herbs as king and bitter and sour herbs as minister. If shaoyang/fire is overruled by taiyang/cold, then medicate with sweet and hot herbs as king and bitter and pungent herbs as minister. If yangming/dryness is overruled by shaoyin/heat, then medicate with pungent and cold herbs as king and bitter and sweet herbs as minister. If taiyang/cold is overruled by shaoyin/heat, then medicate with salty and cold herbs as king and bitter and pungent herbs as minister."

Huang Di asked, "When the ruling influence is extreme and excess as we have discussed in earlier conversations, what do you recommend in terms of treatment?"

Qi Bo replied, "When jueyin/wind is excess, medicate with sweet herbs as king; bitter and pungent herbs as minister; and sour herbs as assistant. When shaoyin/heat is excess, medicate with pungent and cold herbs as king; bitter and salty herbs as minister; and sweet herbs as assistant. When taiyin is excess medicate with salty and hot herbs as king; pungent and sweet herbs as minister; and bitter herbs as assistant. When shaoyang/fire is excess, medicate with pungent and cold herbs as king; sweet and salty herbs as minister; and sweet herbs as assistant. When yangming/dryness is excess, medicate with sour and warming herbs as king; sweet and pungent herbs as minister; and bitter herbs as assistant. Finally, when taiyang/cold is excess, medicate with sweet and hot herbs as king; pungent and sour herbs as minister; and salty herbs as assistant."

Huang Di asked, "Can you please discuss more about the principles governing the art of herbal therapy?"

Qi Bo replied, "In general, mild conditions require a small formula with light-flavored herbs, while acute and severe conditions demand a large formula with thick-flavored herbs. When treating conditions of the upper body one should use more radical herbs while for the lower body gentle herbs would be more appropriate. An herbal decoction should be consumed before meals for conditions located in the lower part of the body, and after meals for conditions in the upper part of the body. One should treat the exterior first when a condition began on the exterior and then attacked the interior. The reverse is true: when a condition originated on the interior and then progressed to the exterior, the interior should be addressed as a priority. Often when a heat condition does not respond after the use of cold or cooling herbs it is because the nature of the illness was not accurately established. Remember: discover the true nature of an illness before embarking on any treatment. Adherence to these general rules will enhance the success of the treatment."

Huang Di asked, "Can you tell me about the three grades of herbs that were recorded in the *Shen Nong Ben Cao* [Shen Nong's Materia Medica]?"

Qi Bo replied, "In ancient times the art of herbology was practiced by categorizing all herbs into three classifications. The first category of herbs was called superior, or immortal, foods because of their lack of side effects and strengthening qualities. These were often incorporated into one's diet and were used as preventive measures. The second category of herbs was called medium or medicinal and were used to rectifying imbalances in the human body. These were used until the patient recovered from their illness and then withdrawn. The third category of herbs was called inferior or radical herbs, so named because they are strong in action and not without side effects; sometimes they are toxic. Therefore these were used often in small amounts and once the desired action took place they were discontinued immediately.

"The paramount mission in healing is to dispel the pathogen and strengthen the patient."

Huang Di said to Qi Bo, "Thank you. This discussion has been most revealing."

CHAPTER 75

THE YELLOW EMPEROR
ON PATHOLOGY

HUANG DI summoned a court adviser, Lei Gong, to his study. "Do you understand the principles of healing?" he asked.

Lei Gong replied, "I have read and studied much. I comprehend these books. But I have difficulty analyzing the true essence of certain things. Clinically speaking, I am not satisfied with my results. My medical knowledge and abilities are quite common. This is not good enough to be of service to the royal family. It is my wish, therefore, for you to teach me how to observe the cosmology of heaven and earth so that I may be an effective instrument in preserving and transmitting the precious wisdom to later generations."

Huang Di said, "Indeed. Do not forget that the myriad things of the universe have an intimate relationship with one another. They may present as varied as yin and yang, internal and external, male and female, upper and lower, but they are all interconnected, interdependent, and intertranscendent. Let us take medicine, for example. As a medical practitioner, one should master the cosmologies of heaven and earth, understand the human mind and spirit, and grasp all sciences of nature. In this way one will have a holistic, integrated perspective, and will grasp the Tao. One can then teach the wisdom and allow it to survive everlastingly. But putting the knowledge in books becomes a precious medium of transmission."

Lei Gong replied, "I am ready."

Huang Di said, "I will teach you from the book called *Yin Yang Zhuan* [Treatise on Yin and Yang]."

Huang Di proceeded, "The qi of the three yang channels protects the body from the outside. It also helps adaptation to environmental changes. However, if the qi flow in the channels is not orderly and rhythmic and becomes rebellious, this will cause internal disharmony. Combined with pathogens from the exterior, this disharmony creates illness, which in turn damages the body's balance of yin and yang."

Lei Gong asked, "What happens when there are disorders in channels simultaneously?"

Huang Di replied, "When the qi of the three yang channels converges suddenly at a specific place, arriving with the speed of a thunderstorm, it is known as 'the compound disorder of the three yang.' In the upper body this causes pathology of the head and neck. In the lower body it causes incontinence of the urine and bowel. This condition does not change in accordance with the general progression of disease. In such cases one cannot properly diagnose whether the condition is in the upper or lower part of the body. *Yin Yang Zhuan* will aid you in the differentiation and analysis of these conditions."

Lei Gong said, "I have much difficulty with this type of disease. My cure rate is quite low. Please enlighten me further."

Huang Di said, "The three yang channels are carriers of yang qi. They are considered yang, or active. But when imbalanced and pathological yang qi converges, one often becomes anxious and easily startled. The onset of the illness is very sudden. As quickly as wind and as violently as thunder, the nine orifices become closed off. The pathogenic yang qi permeates throughout, causing obstruction and dryness of the throat. If it penetrates to the yin area of the lower body, the result is dysentery. When the pathogen traveling in the three yang channels attacks the pericardium and diaphragm directly, one cannot stand up and is relieved by lying down. These conditions are due to invasion by pathogens into the three channels. From this understanding of the three yang, you can begin to understand the relationship of the cosmos with people. You can also differentiate the dynamic interplay of yin and yang, the five elements, and the four seasons."

Lei Gong said, "You have precisely delivered these facts, but my understanding is still shallow. Can you enlighten me further now that I've decided to pursue study of this precious wisdom?"

Huang Di answered, "When learning, one must grasp the core of the teaching. But if one does not understand the true essence of it, one will hesitate and cause confusion. If practitioners of medicine are like these— that is, they have heard the transmission but do not grasp the essence—the wisdom accumulated from many years of human evolution will be lost from the earth forever. So please carry on with diligence."

CHAPTER 76

—

THE IMPORTANCE
OF CORRECT DIAGNOSIS

—

WHILE HUANG Di was in retreat one day he summoned Lei Gong to his study and asked, "You have been diligent in pursuing the knowledge of medicine. I would like to hear about your progress."

Lei Gong replied, "I have studied the medical classic *Mai Jing* [Treatise on Pulse Diagnosis] and in spite of this I am not able to achieve the indicated results with my patients. I do not understand why!"

Huang Di said, "You have in the past demonstrated your comprehension in the pathology of the zang fu organs, acupuncture techniques, and the properties of the materia medica. Now, please be specific as to your uncertainties."

Lei Gong replied, "A condition of heaviness of body and chest discomfort with restlessness can be the symptoms of deficient conditions of either spleen, liver, or kidney. I have administered acupuncture and herbal medicine to patients with these symptoms but have not been effective in all cases. I would like your counsel."

Huang Di answered, "These conditions are not easily differentiated by the common physician because the pulse of a deficient spleen can be floating and weak, mimicking that of the lungs; the pulse of a deficient kidney can be small and floating, like that of the spleen; and the pulse of a deficient liver can be deep, racing, and scattered similar to that of the kidney. This knowledge can be found in the medical classic *Cong Rong* [Treatise on Diagnosis]."

Lei Gong said, "There are those who suffer from heaviness and pain in the head and joints, shortness of breath, timidity, insomnia, abdominal distension, and retching. When I examined their pulses I found it to be floating, wiry, and upon deep palpation hard like a stone. I am perplexed and do not know which organ is the cause."

Huang Di answered, "In nature, pathogenic wind attacks people and invades their bodies. When it stagnates heat is generated, which causes injury to the essence of the viscera. The pathogen, when allowed to linger in the body, mutates and causes various problems. When the pulse shows floating and wiry, it is because the kidney yin has been depleted; when it is sinking and hard like a rock, it is the sign of kidney yang depletion. When the kidneys are disordered, water metabolism becomes impaired and the abdomen becomes distended and discomforting when sleeping at night. The joints become stiff, one becomes timid, and the vitality is low. When the kidney is unable to grasp qi from the lungs, shortness of breath develops. When it is severe the qi rebels and causes retching of clear fluids. As you can see, all the manifestations have their root in the kidney and thus there is no confusion over whether it is spleen or liver."

Lei Gong asked, "There is a patient who suffers from cough, dyspnea, blood in the stools, and extremely weak limbs. I have determined that his lungs are damaged but when I examined his pulses I hesitated about treating him because his pulses were large, floating, and weak. A common physician casually treated him with acupuncture. Afterward, the patient lost more blood in the stools but eventually the bleeding stopped and he recovered. Can you tell me what kind of illness he suffered from?"

Huang Di answered, "Your diagnosis of lung disorder is incorrect in this case. The common physician who seemingly cured the patient did not have a true grasp of the situation. He was merely lucky that the patient recovered from the treatment. You must take note that a superior physician bases his analysis on the fundamental medical principles and considers all factors that are of relevance. Not being attached to convention, he arrives at his conclusion precisely. In this case, the patient's pulse is large, floating, and weak, which signified yang deficiency of the spleen. Since the spleen keeps the blood in the vessels and controls the limbs, the resulting symptoms are extreme weakness of the limbs and extravasation of the blood in the stools. When the yang of the spleen is weak, that is, when the fire is low, water will accumulate in the lungs and cause dyspnea and cough. Therefore, the cause of his illness lies in the spleen and not the lungs.

"Seriously diseased lungs cause disturbances to the qi of the spleen and stomach, resulting in the flight of the essence from all the viscera. Further, vomiting of blood or nosebleed is more likely. You see, it is quite different from a spleen condition.

"Inability to differentiate such conditions reflects the lack of precise learning on the part of the physician. I am responsible for your ignorance, for I was under the impression that you had mastered the medical knowledge. Therefore I am taking this opportunity to cite from the medical classic on diagnosis, *Cong Rong,* in order to help you improve your power of discernment."

Lei Gong arose, bowed and thanked Huang Di for the lesson, then took his leave.

CHAPTER 77

———

THE FIVE FAILINGS
OF PHYSICIANS

———

H UANG DI began by saying, "Alas! The knowledge of life is deep as
an abyss and boundless as the fleeting clouds. The ancient sages practiced medicine by following natural principles combined with their insight-
ful deductions along with the utmost compassion and ethical conduct.
Their way embodies the ideal physician. Do you know, Lei Gong, what
are the five failings and the four virtues regarding a physician?"

Lei Gong arose, bowed respectfully, and replied, "I am young and
ignorant. Will you please enlighten me."

Huang Di nodded and said, "The first failing occurs in diagnosis.
When a physician overlooks factors such as a patient's social and material
status that could contribute to the development of disease, that physician
ends up making an incorrect assessment. A patient who previously held a
respectable social status and enjoyed decadent material existence will most
likely develop illness from internal causes, such as emotional toil, even in
the absence of external pathogens, once he falls from grace and becomes
impoverished. Lack of such observation is a loss to the physician of a valu-
able link that is essential in the accuracy of the diagnosis.

"The second failing occurs in treatment. When a physician neglects a
patient's emotional experiences, which can affect the patient's health
greatly, and indiscriminately tonifies or sedates the patient, the consequence
is further injury to the patient. It is significant to know the patient's lifestyle
and emotional state because emotions such as anger damage the yin, while
overexcitement scatters the yang. Treatment without understanding the
principles of tonification and sedation may cause further exacerbation to a
patient's condition.

"The third failing occurs when the physician lacks deductive reasoning. Much information about a patient's condition is gathered, in addition

to careful observation of the body signs and inquiry of patient's symptoms, from lifestyle, occupation, social and family circumstances, emotional stress, and immediate environment. After gathering the pieces of information, it is the physician's task to utilize to his knowledge and analyze through deduction the entire picture of the patient's illness. Inability to do this limits the physician's effectiveness.

"The fourth failing occurs in counseling. When a physician lacks compassion and sincerity, when a physician is hasty in counseling and does not make the effort to guide the patient's mind and moods in a positive way, that physician has robbed the opportunity to achieve a cure. So much of all illness begins in the mind, and the ability to persuade the patient to change the course of perception and feeling to aid in the healing process is a requirement of a good physician.

"The fifth failing occurs when a physician is simply inept and careless when administering medical care. A physician who is incompetent in medical skills fails to stem the patient's disease from deteriorating. Consequently, when the condition becomes grave, the physician gives a prognosis of death or incurable when the disease actually could have been reversed earlier. This kind of behavior is completely intolerable.

"These five failings form the basis for medical malpractice and are generally due to a physician's superficial grasp of medical principles, techniques, and sociopsychological learning. When the sages practiced medicine, they were certain to have understood the laws of nature and principles of disease, to have mastered diagnosis, to have accomplished techniques of acupuncture and moxibustion, to have been well learned in herbal medicine, and to have attained insights into human relationships and individual temperament. As a result, they delivered their medicine in a thoroughly holistic way.

"The key to effective medicine is to determine the cause and rectify the imbalance of the yuan/original qi of the body. Study the ancient medical classics well. Follow the correct treatment principles and perform your healing with the utmost care and attention. Conduct yourself with the highest virtue and always have compassion toward your patients. In this way you will be outstanding in your cures and never cause malpractice. This is the way of the sage physicians."

CHAPTER 78

THE FOUR LAPSES OF PHYSICIANS

H UANG DI received Lei Gong in the Great Hall and asked, "You have studied all the important medical classics and you have had much experience in medical practice. Tell me about your successes and failures and the reasons behind them."

Lei Gong answered, "I have practiced by following the principles of the classics and performed techniques taught by my teachers, but clinically my results are still far from satisfactory. Why is this?"

Huang Di replied, "It is because you are young and inexperienced. It is also because you have allowed some anecdotes you have heard to confuse your analytical perception. When a physician is unable to attain consistent cures it is often because of a lack of focus in the evaluation and analysis of the patient's outwardly manifested symptoms and signs and inwardly generated pathology. Therefore, he or she hesitates and makes mistakes.

"A lack of understanding in the transmutation of yin and yang in diagnosis is the first blunder of a physician.

"Administering medicine without proficiency in knowledge and skills, thereby causing injury to patients, is the second blunder of a physician.

"Ineptitude in the investigation into the etiology of an illness by neglecting to take into consideration the patient's social and material circumstances, immediate environment, dietary habits, emotional tendencies, and possible toxic contaminations constitutes the third blunder of a physician.

"Being boastful of lucky cures, falsely exaggerating the nature of an illness, haste and carelessness in one's action, and disparagement of the reputation of the teacher are the traits that comprise the fourth blunder of a physician."

Huang Di turned to Lei Gong and reflectively remarked, "Alas! The way of healing is so profound. It is deep as the oceans and boundless as the skies. How many truly know it?"

CHAPTER 79

THE THREE YIN AND THREE YANG CHANNELS IN THE HUMAN BODY

—

O N the first day of spring, Huang Di observed the weather of nature and then turned to ask Lei Gong, "Based on the principles of yin and yang and the channels, which channel do you think is primary in the circulation of qi?"

Lei Gong replied, "The seventy-two days of spring is the beginning of the four seasons. It corresponds to the element wood, the color green, and the organ liver. Hence, I think the liver and its channel are the primary ones."

Huang Di shook his head and said, "On the contrary, according to the ancient classics, what you mentioned is the secondary in the energetic order." He then sent Lei Gong away.

After fasting and bathing, Lei Gong returned to the Great Hall ready to receive further teachings.

Huang Di said, "The qi of the five zang organs circulates throughout the body in a continuous fashion, like the universe with its myriad galaxies. The qi flow begins in the taiyang/bladder and small intestine channels, which serve as the primordial, dynamic beginning spreading along the back of the trunk and the limbs. It is regarded sometimes as the father. The qi then flows onwards to the yangming/stomach and large intestine channels, which act as the defender as it traverses the front of the trunk and the limbs. Next the qi travels through the shaoyang/gallbladder and sanjiao channels on the sides of the trunk and limbs. It is the bridge between the interior and the exterior of the body, or where the qi makes its entry into the deeper yin environment.

"The first yin channels the qi passes through are the taiyin/spleen and lung channels, which are the outermost channels amongst the yin channels. The taiyin channels are the great nurturer, sometimes regarded as the mother. The qi winds its way further into the shaoyin/kidney and heart channels, which are the gatherer of qi into the deep reservoir of the body. As the qi penetrates into its final destination, before it begins the cycle all over again, it arrives at the jueyin/liver and pericardium channels. The yin at its peak starts to decline, allowing the yang to rise, like the moon, which is symbolic of yin in the night sky. When the night is dying, the sun, which is symbolic of yang, will be born. The jueyin channels are the extreme yin vessels which act as transition between yin and yang as the qi flows harmoniously through them, maintaining a delicate balance. The cycle is repeated, always following this order, unless there is pathology, which can disrupt the flow of qi."

Lei Gong appeared unsure and said, "I still do not completely grasp the significance of the three yin and the three yang channels."

Huang Di continued, "The condition of the three yin and the three yang channels can be detected at the radial pulse. The pulse of the afflicted taiyang channel will express as floating and tense. When the yangming channel is affected, its pulse displays wiry, rapid, and sinking qualities. However, if the same pulse is present in severe febrile disease, death may be imminent. If the shaoyang channel is imbalanced, it will typically show a wiry, rapid, and suspended pulse, both at the radial and at the carotid positions. In the event that the decaying pulse of the shaoyang channel appears, death will shortly ensue.

"In taiyin channel disorders the pulse will sink and become hidden and hard to detect. In this case the qi has prolapsed and is unable to ascend. When the shaoyin channel is dysfunctional it manifests pulses similar to that of the taiyin channel. And finally, when the jueyin is diseased critically, its pulse will be floating, slippery, flooding, and suspended without anchor. This indicates danger and the impending collapse of qi."

Lei Gong nodded in acknowledgement and said, "I have now finally begun to grasp the diagnostic value of these channels. But I would like to learn still more about their pathology."

Huang Di said, "When the yangming and jueyin channels are diseased with the yangming channel being the primary, its pulse will become soft and moving and the qi will be obstructed at the orifices. When the taiyang and jueyin channels are diseased with the taiyang channels the primary one, its pulse will be excessive, reflecting the uncontrollable water flooding the body and disabling the five zang organs. Outward signs are terror and fright. When the shaoyin and yangming channels are diseased with the origin in the lungs, the shaoyin pulse will be sinking, reflecting weakening of the lungs and the spleen as well as problems to the extremities. If the origin is in the kidneys, the patient will present manic tendencies. When the shaoyin and shaoyang channels are diseased, the kidneys lose control of water metabolism, leading to the accumulation of pathogenic yin in the epigastrium and the obstruction of the flow of the yang qi. The pores will not open and no sweat will occur. The extremities will feel as if they are separated from the trunk. In compound conditions of the jueyin and shaoyang channels, wood is excessive and overacts on the earth if the pulse is intermittent and dying. Its manifestations are also unpredictable; sometimes in the upper body it shows dry and irritated throat, sometimes in the lower body one finds lack of appetite and frequent diarrhea. In compound conditions of the yangming and taiyin channels, tumor is the result when there is a lack of intercourse between the yin and the yang, with the yang qi stagnating in the exterior, while suppurative skin lesions are the results of yin qi stagnating in the interior. If the stagnation occurs in the lower abdomen, disease of the genitals would be the outcome.

"When you have fully grasped the principles of the three yin and three yang channels, you will then know which channel and organ is the primary and which is the secondary, and you will be able to translate the transmutations of disease among the channels."

Lei Gong asked, "Can you talk about the reasons behind why some illnesses result in quick death?"

Huang Di answered, "If an illness occurs in the three months of winter displaying signs of excess of heat, as well as signs of decaying pulse by the first month of spring, the patient will not survive beyond early summer as the yang of nature reaches the zenith. In another illness of the same period though displaying signs of decaying pulse in the winter, the patient will not make it past the first month of spring, when nature is just beginning to stir. If an illness occurs in the three months of spring and a decaying pulse is detected, the patient will surely die along with the withering of the vegetation at the end of the fall. If an illness occurs in the three months of summer, with spleen involvement and signs of decaying pulse present, the patient shall not live beyond ten more days; and if signs of chaos of yin and yang are present in the pulses, the patient will have difficulty seeing the harvest full moon in the eighth month. If an illness of the taiyang channel occurs in the three months of autumn, the condition will be rectified naturally even in the absence of medical care. However, if the yin and yang are dissociated, the patient will have difficulty standing and sitting. If in the same period the decaying pulse of the taiyang channel is detected, the patient will pass on when the water freezes in the winter. If the decaying pulse of shaoyin is present the patient's death will be around the first rain in the spring."

CHAPTER 80

—

GROWTH AND DECLINE
OF ENERGY

—

LEI GONG inquired, "The energy of a person can be excessive or deficient. Can you elaborate on the normal and the abnormal flow of this energy?"

Huang Di answered, "Normally, the yang qi flows upward on the left and the yin qi flows downward on the right. In the elderly, the qi flows upward because of the deficiency in the lower body. In the youthful, the qi flows downward because of the abundance in the lower body. Seasonally, the spring and summer are characterized by an abundance of yang while the autumn and winter are characterized by yin. These are natural and normal conditions. If on the contrary the natural orders are reversed, where during the spring and summer yin predominates while during the autumn and winter yang dominates, these phenomena are abnormal and can lead to destruction."

Lei Gong asked, "Will destruction still occur even in situations of abundance instead of deficiency?"

Huang Di replied, "Yes. For example, when excess qi is impeded in the upper body and unable to descend, it will cause vertex headache and severe cold blockage with icy-cold legs. If this occurs in the youthful during the autumn or winter, death is certain. If it occurs in the elderly during the same seasons the prognosis is favorable.

"If a blockage is caused by insufficiency of qi the patient will suffer from nightmares and, in some instances, delirium. The pulses of the three yang and the three yin channels will display suspended and floating as well as thin and faint qualities, respectively.

"People's dreams will often reflect their state of energy. When the lung qi is deficient one will dream of white objects and murderous events, while if it is in an excessive state one dreams of battles in action. When the kidney qi is deficient one will dream of drowning, while if it is in an excessive state one dreams of hiding underwater with extreme terror. When the liver qi is deficient one will dream of fragrance of flowers, while if it is in an excessive state one dreams of hiding behind a large tree. When the heart qi is deficient one will dream of putting out fire, while if it is in an excessive state one dreams of a large barn fire. When the spleen qi is deficient one will dream of starvation, while if it is in an excessive state one dreams of construction of a wall or building. These dreams usually come from either a deficiency of yin qi or an excess of yang qi of each individual zang organ and can be useful as diagnostic clues.

"In diagnosis there are five areas that deserve close examination. They are the pulses, the channels that correspond to the organs, the muscles, the tendons, and the acupoints. In general, close scrutiny of these five areas will provide sufficient information to make a proper diagnosis; however, there are cases that display inconsistent pulse patterns, making accurate diagnosis difficult. In this situation, one must inquire and investigate in depth about the patient's social and material existence, immediate environment, emotional tendencies, past history, and anything else that may contribute to a correct diagnosis of the patient's condition.

"When a physician encounters an excess condition, that physician must also look for what is deficient as well. Specifically, poor prognosis is given when a patient displays degeneration in outward signs and symptoms and pulses, or degeneration in only the pulses and not the signs and symptoms. However, as long as the pulses of the patient remain strong, even if the signs and symptoms are grave, the prognosis is favorable.

"A physician needs to possess a moral conscience, ethical conduct, and a compassionate attitude toward those in need of attention. In all interactions with patients the physician is always composed, takes the necessary time, remains objective, and performs every procedure with the utmost care and precision. In diagnosis, all the available facts and probes are gathered for the hidden facts through keen observation, olfaction and listening, inquiry and palpation. When the facts are collected, that knowledge and experience are combined with logical deduction and penetrating insights to arrive at the correct diagnosis. Treatments are then administered with equal effectiveness. At all times the physician is concentrated and does not allow distractions. In violation of these maxims a physician cannot expect to last long in the medical profession and continue to help others and thus defeat the original virtuous purpose of entering that profession."

CHAPTER 81

—

SUBTLE REASONING

—

I N the Great Hall sat Huang Di and his attendants. Lei Gong remarked, "I have been teaching others the medical arts and found that some of my students are not quick to grasp and their clinical results are also not satisfactory. Having received additional teaching from you I have passed on to them the essential medical principles and emphasized the importance of gathering facts from a patient's past history, lifestyle, social and material existence, emotional tendencies, seasonal exposure, and other considerations so that a complete picture can emerge and a thorough understanding can transpire for them. Today, I am embarrassed to ask you a minor question that is not addressed in the medical classics."

Huang Di responded, "Indeed, the medical art is immense and difficult to fathom in every detail."

Lei Gong asked, "Why are there people who are grief-stricken but do not shed tears, or others who have tears but are not sad?"

Huang Di replied, "This knowledge is basic and can be found in the medical classics. The eyes correspond to the liver, but it is the heart that manifests its shen/spirit through the eyes. The tears are the jin ye/body fluids that are governed by the kidneys. When one engages emotionally the shen is stirred, the perception becomes blurry, and the kidneys lose control of fluid, the tears. Additionally, the head contains the sea of marrow that is also governed by the kidneys, which react in concert by discharging a fluid out of the nasal passageway.

"When one is grief-stricken and cannot shed tears it is either because the disturbed shen causes the qi to rush to the head area and results in obstruction of the tear ducts, or because the shen remained rational and undisturbed and caused no reaction from the kidneys. There are others who shed tears without emotional disturbance. These instances are usually due to exposure to wind pathogens or excess heat in the head area. This is like nature; on the heels of a hot spell the wind stirs and rain will usually follow."

BIBLIOGRAPHY

CHINESE PUBLICATIONS BEFORE 1911

Gao Shi Zhong. *Suwen Zhi Jie* (Genuine Explanation of the Yellow Emperor's Simple Questions). 1693 (Qing).

Hu Shu. *Huang Di Neijing Suwen Xiao Yi* (Annotated Neijing: Simple Questions). 1880 (Qing).

Hua Bo Ren. *Du Suwen Cao* (Commentaries on *Simple Questions*). 1355 (Yuan).

Li Nien Yi. *Neijing Zhi Yao* (Essentials of *The Yellow Emperor's Classic*). 1642 (Ming).

Lin Yi. *Xin Jiao Zheng* (Revision of *Simple Questions*). 1057 (Song).

Liu Wan Su. *Suwen Xuan Ji Yuan Bing Lun* (Standards of the Mysterious Inner Workings of the Origin of Illness Discussed in *Simple Questions*). 1186 (Song).

Ma Zhong Hua. *Suwen Zhu Zheng Fa Wei* (Explanation of the Yellow Emperor's Classic Syndrome Complex). 1586 (Ming).

Tao Zhi. *Suwen Jing Jie Jie* (Analysis of the *Simple Questions*). 1677 (Qing).

Wang Bing. *Bu Zhu Huang Di Neijing Suwen* (Revised and Elucidated *Yellow Emperor's Classic*: Simple Questions). 762 (Tang).

Wu Kun. *Suwen Wu Zhu* (Wu's Explanations of *Simple Questions*). 1594 (Ming).

Yang Shang Shan. *Huang Di Neijing Taisu* (Simple Questions: The Yellow Emperor's Classic). 605 (Sui).

Zhang Qi. *Suwen Shi Yi* (Explanation of *Simple Questions*). 1830 (Qing).

Zhang Zhi Cong. *Suwen Zhi Zhu* (Explanations of the Complete *Simple Questions*). 1672 (Qing).

Zhou Xue Hai. *Neijing Ping Wen* (Analysis of *The Yellow Emperor's Classic*). 1896 (Qing).

PUBLICATIONS AFTER 1911

Academy of Traditional Chinese Medicine (TCM) and the Guangdong College of TCM, eds. *Dictionary of Traditional Chinese Medical Terms and Nomenclature*. Beijing: People's Health Press, 1973.

Beijing College of TCM. *A Textbook of the Yellow Emperor's Classic*. Beijing: Medical and Hygiene Press, 1975.

Beijing Medical College. *Dictionary of Traditional Chinese Medicine*. Hong Kong: Commercial Press, 1984.

Beijing Institute of TCM. *Explanation of the Yellow Emperor's Classic*. Shanghai: Science and Technology Press, 1964.

Cheng, S., and J. Meng, eds. *Explanation of the Yellow Emperor's Classic*. Shanghai: Shanghai Science and Technology Press, 1984.

Fang, Y., and J. Shu, eds. *Explanation of Phase Energetics of the Yellow Emperor's Classic: The Simple Questions.* Beijing: People's Health Press, 1984.

Gansu School of Public Health. *Explanation of Common TCM Terms.* Gansu: People's Press, 1975.

Guo, Hecun, ed. *Annotated Yellow Emperor's Classic: Simple Questions.* Tianjin: Tianjin Science and Technology Press, 1981.

Kaptchuk, Ted. *The Web That Has No Weaver.* New York: Congdon and Weed, 1983.

Nanjing College of TCM. *Explanation of the Yellow Emperor's Classic: The Simple Questions.* Shanghai: Shanghai Science and Technology Press, 1959.

——. *Explanation of the Yellow Emperor's Classic.* Shanghai: Shanghai Science and Technology Press, 1978.

Ni, Hua-Ching. *The Book of Changes and the Unchanging Truth,* rev. ed. Santa Monica: SevenStar Communications, 1993.

——. *Tao, the Subtle Universal Law and the Integral Way of Life.* Santa Monica: SevenStar Communications, 1993.

Ou, Ming. *Chinese-English Glossary of Common Terms in Traditional Chinese Medicine.* Hong Kong: Joint Publishing Co., 1982.

Porkert, Manfred. *The Theoretical Foundation of Chinese Medicine.* M.I.T. East Asian Science Series, vol. 3. Cambridge: MIT Press, 1974.

Qin, Bowei. *The Essence of the Yellow Emperor's Classic.* Beijing: People's Health Press, 1957.

Shandong College of TCM and Research Institute of TCM Literature. *Wu Kun's Interpretation of the Yellow Emperor's Classic: Simple Questions.* Shandong: Shandong Science and Technology Press, 1984.

Shandong Research Institute of TCM. *Vernacular Explanation of the Yellow Emperor's Classic.* Shandong Science and Technology Press, 1979.

Sichuang Research Institute of TCM. *Annotated Interpretation of the Yellow Emperor's Classic: The Simple Questions and the Difficult Questions.* Sichuang: Sichuang Science and Technology Press, 1987.

TCM Research Institute and Guangdong Institute of TCM. *Selected Explanation of TCM Terms.* Beijing: People's Press, 1973.

Unschuld, Paul U. *Medicine in China: A History of Ideas.* Los Angeles: University of California Press, 1985.

Wang, Qi, ed. *Subject Studies of the Yellow Emperor's Classic.* Shandong: Shandong Science and Technology Press, 1985.

Wang, Qi, et al., eds. *Modern Interpretations of the Yellow Emperor's Classic: Simple Questions.* Guizhou: Guizhou People's Press, 1981.

Xu, Zhenlin. *Phase Energetics of the Yellow Emperor's Classic.* Shanghai: Shanghai Science and Technology Literary Press, 1990.

Yue, Q., W. Yu, and Z. Liu, eds. *New Explanation of the Yellow Emperor's Classic.* Sichuan: Sichuan People's Press, 1980.

Zhou, S., and J. Chen, eds. *Essentials of the Yellow Emperor's Classic.* Gansu: Gansu People's Press, 1982.

Zhou, F., W. Wang, and G. Xu, eds. *Vernacular Explanation of the Yellow Emperor's Classic: Simple Questions.* Beijing: People's Health Press, 1958.

ABOUT THE TRANSLATOR

Author, lecturer, and licensed practitioner of Traditional Chinese Medicine, Mao-shing Ni, Ph.D., D.O.M., is the cofounder and vice president of Yo San University of Traditional Chinese Medicine in Santa Monica, California, where he has trained many medical professionals. Born and raised in a family medical tradition that spans many generations, Dr. Ni studied Chinese medicine and Taoist arts and science with his father, the renowned physician and author Hua-Ching Ni, and also received advanced training in China and the United States.

Maoshing Ni has lectured and taught workshops throughout the country on such diverse subjects as longevity, preventive medicine, Chinese therapeutic nutrition, Chinese herbal medicine, physiognomy (facial reading), Feng Shui (geomancy), acupuncture, T'ai Chi, Qi Gong, stress management, and the history of medicine.

Dr. Ni is also president of Traditions of Tao, a company that researches and produces longevity herbal food products. Most recently he is a member of the editorial board for the encyclopedic book *Alternative Medicine: A Definitive Guide* and the monthly *Alternative Medicine Digest*. Currently he maintains a full-time medical practice with his brother, Dr. Daoshing Ni, in Santa Monica, California.

INDEX